Titles of related interest

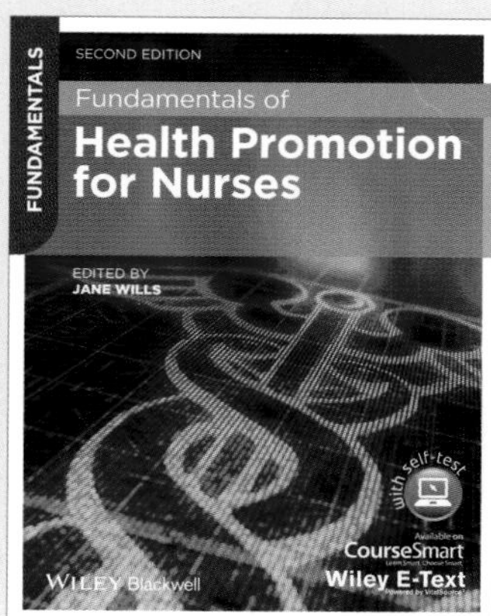

ISBN: 978-1-118-51577-8

Review of the 1st edition:
'This is a really useful text. Health promotion, an essential aspect of the nurse's role, has not previously been given sufficient prominence. The chapters are written by notable authors and despite their diversity, there is continuity to it, giving it an overall coherence and sense of whole. This is a thoroughly useful text.' Nursing Times

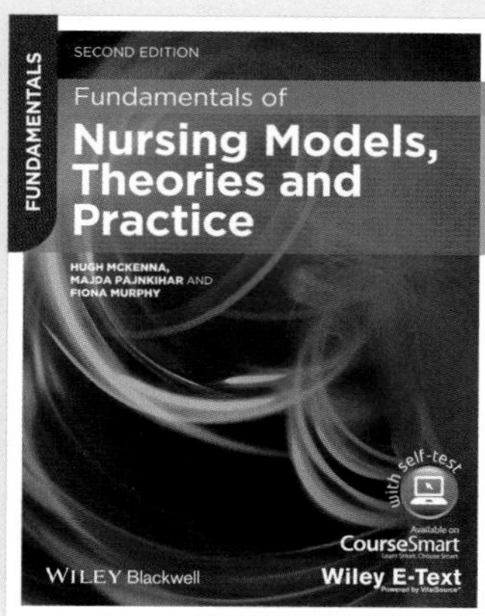

ISBN: 978-0-470-65776-8

Review of the 1st edition:
'A very practical & focused book. Well supported by existing theory' (Nursing lecturer, University of Hertfordshire)

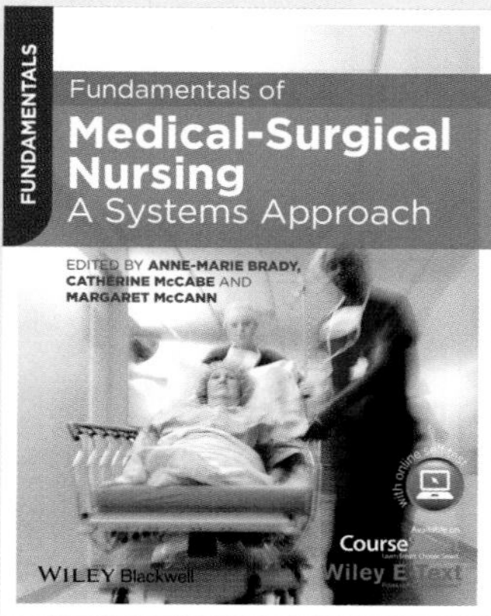

ISBN : 978-0-470-65823-9

'A serious contender for the position of 'key course text' for most adult branch courses running in the UK.' (Lecturer in Adult Nursing, Bangor University)

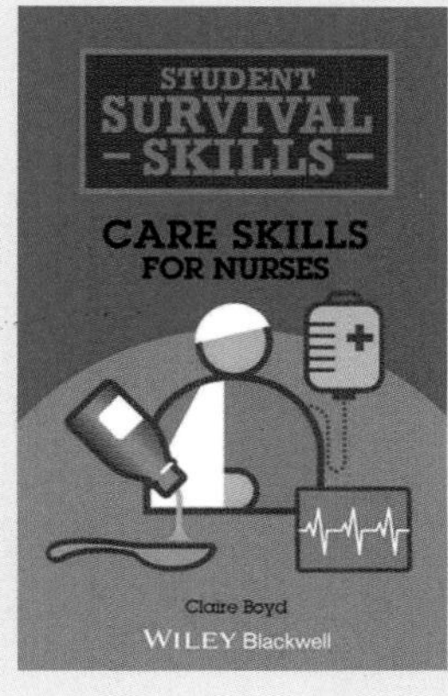

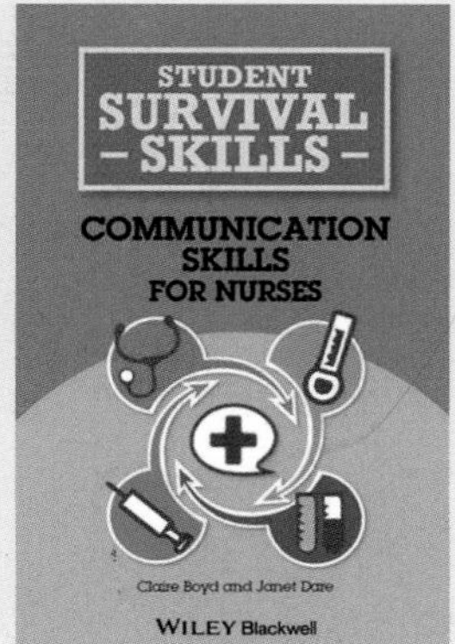

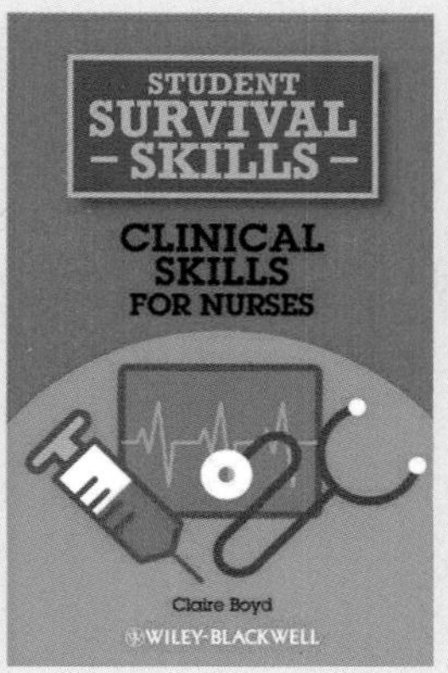

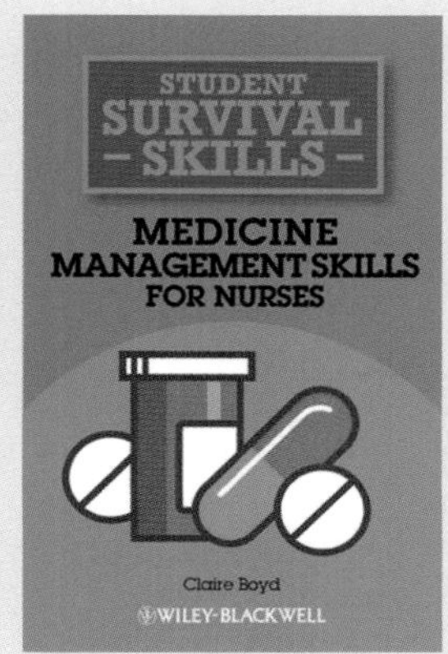

ISBN: 978-1-118-65738-6 ISBN: 978-1-118-76752-8 ISBN: 978-1-118-44877-9 ISBN: 978-1-118-44885-4

'I love this series…I can't wait to get my hands on them' (Second year nursing student, University of Abertay, Dundee)

Fundamentals of

Palliative Care for Student Nurses

This book is dedicated to all the patients and families we have been privileged to work with during our careers; with immense gratitude for all that they taught us.

FIRST EDITION

Fundamentals of Palliative Care for Student Nurses

Authored by Megan Rosser and Helen C Walsh, with contributions from Chantal Patel

MEGAN ROSSER

Director for CPD/Non Professional Undergraduate Programmes, College of Human and Health Sciences, Swansea University

AND

HELEN C. WALSH

Senior lecturer, College of Human and Health Sciences, Swansea University

WILEY Blackwell

Registered office: John Wiley & Sons, Ltd, The Atrium, Southern Gate, Chichester, West Sussex, PO19 8SQ, UK

Editorial offices: 9600 Garsington Road, Oxford, OX4 2DQ, UK

The Atrium, Southern Gate, Chichester, West Sussex, PO19 8SQ, UK
111 River Street, Hoboken, NJ 07030-5774, USA

For details of our global editorial offices, for customer services and for information about how to apply for permission to reuse the copyright material in this book please see our website at www.wiley.com/wiley-blackwell

Library of Congress *Cataloging-in-Publication* Data

Fundamentals of palliative care for student nurses / edited by Megan Rosser, Helen Walsh.
p. ; cm.
Includes bibliographical references and index.
ISBN 978-1-118-43780-3 (pbk.)
I. Rosser, Megan, editor. II. Walsh, Helen, 1957- editor.
[DNLM: 1. Nursing Care--methods. 2. Palliative Care--methods. 3. Terminal Care--methods. WY 152.3]
R726.8
616.02'9--dc23

2014004008

A catalogue record for this book is available from the British Library.

Wiley also publishes its books in a variety of electronic formats. Some content that appears in print may not be available in electronic books.

Set in 10/12 pt Myriad Pro by Laserwords Private Limited
Printed and bound in Singapore by Markono Print Media Pte Ltd

1 2014

Contents

About the series

Wiley's *Fundamentals* series are a wide-ranging selection of textbooks written to support pre-registration nursing and other healthcare students throughout their course. Packed full of useful features such as learning objectives, activities to test knowledge and understanding, and clinical scenarios, the titles are also highly illustrated and fully supported by interactive MCQs, and each one includes access to a **Wiley E-Text: powered by VitalSource** – an interactive digital version of the book including downloadable text and images and highlighting and note-taking facilities. Accessible on your laptop, mobile phone or tablet device, the *Fundamentals series* is *the* most flexible, supportive textbook series available for nursing and healthcare students today.

The Authors

Megan Rosser RGN, DN cert, BSc (Hons) MSc (London) PG Cert Learning and Teaching

Megan began her nursing career at Charing Cross Hospital and qualified as a Registered General Nurse in 1985. Since then she has specialised in oncology and in palliative care, spending time in her early clinical years at the Royal Marsden and St. Francis Hospice Romford. The last 7 years of her clinical practice were spent as a community Macmillan nurse in West Essex. Megan moved into education in 1999 and worked at St. Christopher's Hospice, Kings College London and the Macmillan National Institute for Education before moving to Swansea 10 years ago. Megan is currently the Director for continuing professional development in the College of Human and Health Sciences at Swansea University and has previously published in the areas of cancer nursing, palliative care, action research, transition experiences, mentorship and evidence based practice.

Helen C Walsh SRN, RM, RHV, Dip HE Business Administration, MSc, PGCert Education

Helen started her nursing career at the Royal Masonic Hospital and qualified as a State registered Nurse in 1979. After a brief spell working in Urology Helen trained as a midwife and then pursued a career in cardio-thoracic nursing for 3.5 years. After training as a health visitor Helen moved into the area of palliative care nursing, working in a number of increasingly senior posts at St. David's Foundation in Newport before taking up the post of Senior Macmillan Nurse at Ty Olwen Palliative Care Service in Swansea. Helen moved into nurse education in 2005 and is currently a senior lecturer in the College of Human and Health Sciences at Swansea University, her particular areas of interest include communication, clinical supervision, portfolio development and learning through patchwork texts. Helen has previously published works in the areas of palliative care and bereavement care and has presented at a number of conferences.

Acknowledgements

Megan would like to thank her partner Sue Waite for her unfailing belief, support and encouragement.

Helen would like to acknowledge Jen and Fran for their support, encouragement and love.

Preface

The aim of palliative care is to improve the quality of life of people living with serious chronic illnesses such as cancer, cardiac failure, Alzheimer's disease and renal failure. Traditionally, palliative care was considered only to be needed by patients living with cancer but thankfully it has long been acknowledged that palliative care should be available to all people in need, regardless of their diagnosis. Palliative care is holistic care and addresses people's physiological, social, emotional and spiritual needs as well as their physical needs. Good fundamental 'general palliative care' can be provided by any knowledgeable health care professional; relatively few people require specialist palliative care provided by specialist teams.

Whilst primarily aimed at student nurses, it is our belief that this book also contains useful information for registered nurses who wish to learn more about palliative care. This book seeks to provide you with an introduction to the main principles and theories of palliative care in order to give you the basic essential knowledge to enhance your confidence in caring for people with palliative care needs. The first section of the book introduces you to the development of palliative care practice, focussing on the underpinning principles; the second section considers how these principles apply in clinical situations in order to achieve optimal care and quality of life for patients and their families. The third and final section focuses on your continued development in the practice of palliative care.

In keeping with the philosophical approach of the series we have tried to make the book as interactive as possible. Throughout the book there are a number of activities for you to undertake, encouraging you to take time out from reading to think about your current practice and to consider how new knowledge gained from this book might develop your nursing care. In order to help you apply the information in the book to your own practice we have tried to give clinical examples wherever possible; there are patient scenarios in most chapters. There are opportunities at the end of many chapters to test your learning and the companion website presents short MCQs for each chapter to enable further self-assessment of learning.

The term patient is used throughout the text in preference to 'service user', 'client' or 'consumer' because of familiarity and ease of use. Whilst the term 'patient' may have negative connotations for some health care professionals it is still the most commonly used term and the most easily understood and is therefore felt by us to be the most appropriate. True patient centred palliative care should overcome the imbalances of power perceived by some to be associated with the term patient.

About the companion website

This book is accompanied by a companion website:

www.wiley.com/go/rosser_walsh/fundamentals_of_palliative_care

The website includes:

- Interactive MCQs for self-assessment
- Useful online resources

I

The principles of palliative care

1

The development of palliative care

Introduction

This chapter explores the history and development of palliative care from the early days of the hospice movement through to the development of specialist palliative care and end of life care. It will track the extension of palliative care beyond cancer diagnosis, which is underpinned by the principle of provision of care according to need, not diagnosis. The differences between palliative care and other areas of care will be explored. The provision of palliative care for patients in minority groups is considered as well as the policies and strategies that have shaped the development of the speciality.

Learning outcomes

By the end of this chapter you will be able to

- identify key events in the development of hospice and palliative care;
- describe palliative care and specialist palliative care;

(*continued*)

Fundamentals of Palliative Care for Student Nurses, First Edition. Megan Rosser and Helen C. Walsh.

Companion website: www.wiley.com/go/rosser_walsh/fundamentals_of_palliative_care

Learning outcomes *(continued)*

- identify the key principles of palliative care;
- discuss the provision of palliative care across care settings;
- discuss the extension of palliative care services beyond cancer diagnosis;
- discuss some of the challenges facing hard-to-reach groups requiring palliative care.

What is palliative care?

Simply put, palliative care 'focuses on the relief of pain and other symptoms and problems experienced in serious illness. The goal of palliative care is to improve quality of life, by increasing comfort, promoting dignity and providing a support system to the person who is ill and those close to them.' (dying matters 2012).

Since the development of St Christopher's hospice in 1967, the growth of palliative care has been driven by charities, health care providers and government policy. The significant early developments and key policies are presented in Figures 1.1 and 1.2.

Cicely Saunders the founder of the modern day hospice movement was driven by a profound Christian faith and a fundamental belief that 'You matter because you are you, and you

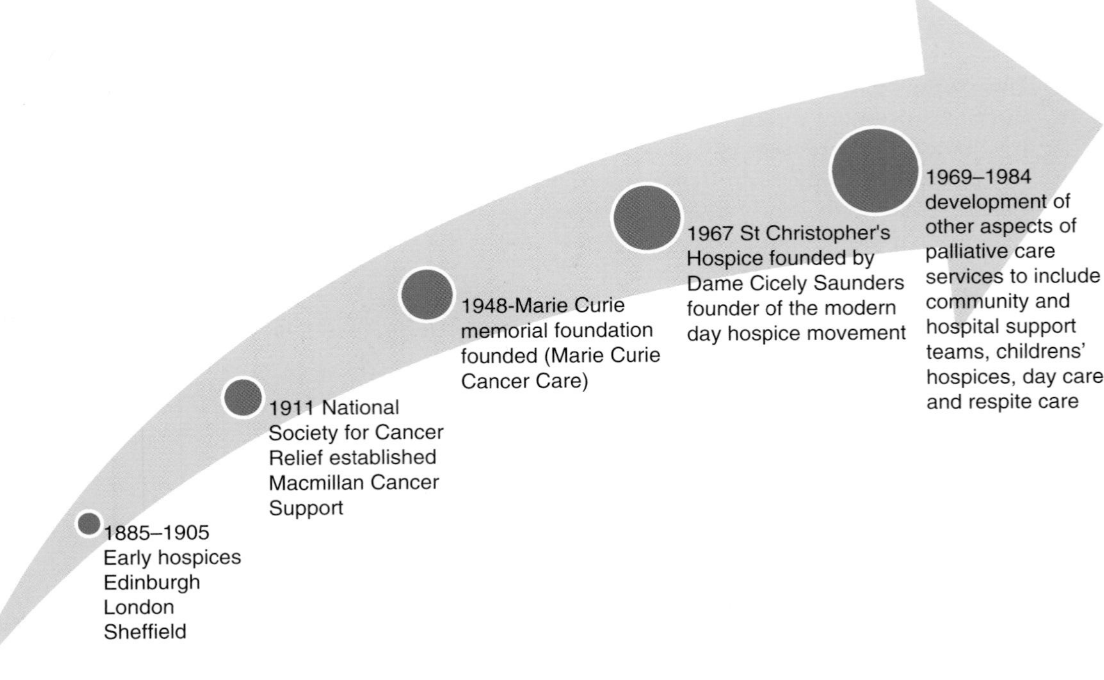

Figure 1.1 The early development of palliative care services in the United Kingdom.

1995
• Calman-Hine Report
1997
• Introduction of Liverpool Care Pathway (LCP)
2001
• Pilot of the Gold Standards Framework
2002
• Preferred place of care documentation
2004
• NICE Improving supportive and palliative care for adults with cancer
2005
• National Service Framework for Long Term Conditions
2008
• End of Life Care Strategy
2013
• Review and recommended phasing out of LCP in England

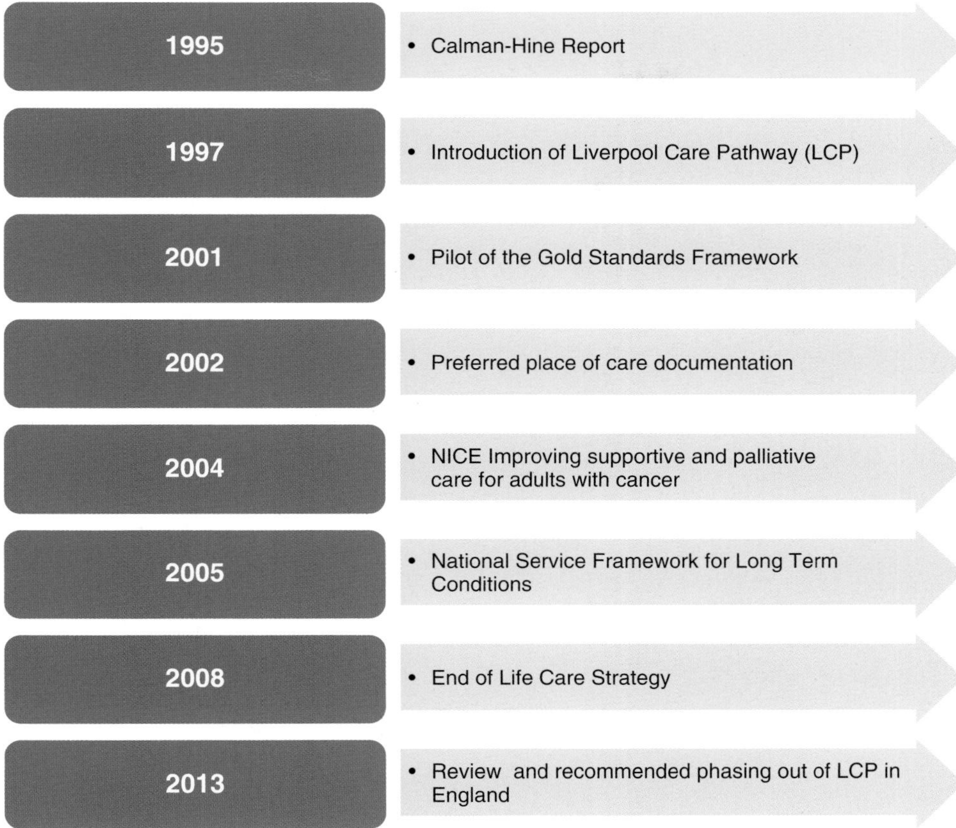

Figure 1.2 Key policy developments in palliative care in the United Kingdom.

matter to the last moment of your life'. Whilst the influence of religion has diminished over time the central belief of the value of people is paramount to palliative care. Today there are over 200 inpatient units and palliative care is provided in a number of other care settings, including hospitals, the community and day care centres. Most hospices are independent, local charities, only receiving a minority of their funding from the NHS.

There are a number of definitions relating to the provision of palliative care and each is discussed in the following text.

Supportive care

Palliative care has come to be regarded as part of supportive care formally introduced by the National Institute for Clinical Excellence (NICE) in 2004. Supportive care describes all care provided to patients, friends and family throughout their illness, including the time before diagnosis has been reached, when patients may be undergoing a number of investigations. The aim of supportive care is to help the patients and their families to cope with their condition and treatment. It helps the patient to maximise the benefits of treatment and to live as well

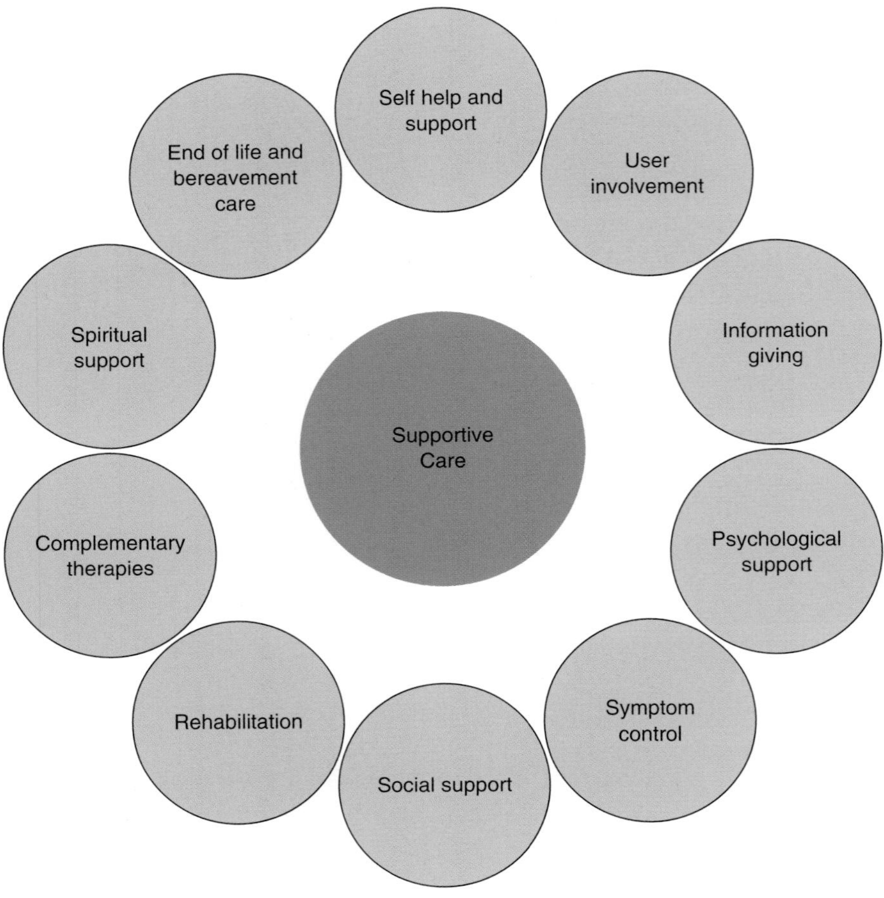

Figure 1.3 The components of supportive care.

as possible with the effects of the disease (National Council for Palliative Care (NCPC) 2010). Figure 1.3 shows the components of supportive care.

Palliative care

Palliative care is defined in Fact Box 1.1.

Fact Box 1.1

The World Health Organization (WHO) (2014) defines palliative care as:

'an approach that improves the quality of life of patients and their families facing the problems associated with life-threatening illness, through the prevention and relief of suffering by means of early identification and impeccable assessment and treatment of pain and other problems, physical, psychosocial and spiritual.

The WHO principles of palliative care are listed in Fact Box 1.2:

Fact Box 1.2

The principles of palliative care

WHO principles of palliative care

- provides relief from pain and other distressing symptoms;
- affirms life and regards dying as a normal process;
- intends neither to hasten nor postpone death;
- integrates the psychological and spiritual aspects of patient care;
- offers a support system to help patients live as actively as possible until death;
- offers a support system to help the family cope during the patient's illness and in their own bereavement;
- uses a team approach to address the needs of patients and their families, including bereavement counselling, if indicated;
- will enhance quality of life, and may also positively influence the course of illness;
- is applicable early in the course of illness, in conjunction with other therapies that are intended to prolong life, such as chemotherapy or radiation therapy, and includes those investigations needed to better understand and manage distressing clinical complications.

These principles highlight an holistic, humanistic approach to caring for the whole person throughout their illness, rather than focusing on the disease or condition. Palliative care responds to the changing needs of the patient and family over time, recognising that the disease progression and the associated experiences are unique to each person.

Specialist palliative care

As the palliative care movement developed and grew there was an expressed need to differentiate between palliative care and specialist palliative care to ensure that patients and their families were receiving the most appropriate care. It was acknowledged that a minority of people with complex needs would require direct or indirect input from specialist teams, identified as 'those services with palliative care as their core speciality with a high level of professional skills from trained staff and a high staff: patient ratio' (NCHSPCS, 1995).

Once the differences between palliative and specialist palliative care had been established there was an expectation that everyone living with a life-threatening illness was entitled to receive appropriate palliative care regardless of health setting; therefore, each health professional has a duty to practice the palliative care approach as an integral component of good clinical practice, referring to specialist palliative practitioners when necessary (NCHSPCS, 1997).

End of life care

As the meaning of palliative care has developed beyond care provided for those who are dying it became necessary to coin a new definition – 'end of life care'. This is acknowledged by the Department of Health (2008) as care that helps all those with advanced, progressive, incurable illness to live as well as possible until they die. It enables the supportive and palliative care needs of both patient and family to be identified and met throughout the last phase of life and into bereavement.

Where is palliative care provided?

Palliative care services have extended far beyond the hospices of the early movement (Figure 1.4).

As stated by NCHSPCS (1997) fundamental palliative care should be provided by the patient's primary carers, be it the ward teams or the district nurses or GPs. Specialist palliative care practitioners may be involved in the management of more challenging situations such as complex pain or symptom problems or complex psychological needs or family dynamics. Specialist practitioners should withdraw once the problem has settled or if the patient is admitted for specialist palliative care. Nowadays, hospices are used for specialist palliative care rather than respite, which was not the case in the early days. Respite is often provided by nursing homes, or by Marie Curie nurses who provide periods of respite overnight or during the day in the patient's home. Hospice at home teams may become involved towards the very end of the patient's life to enable them to die at home.

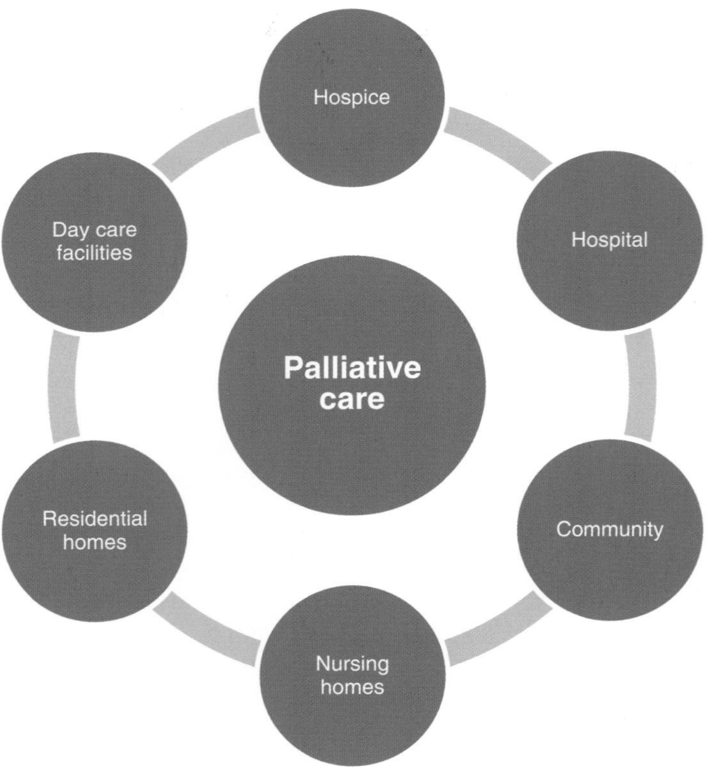

Figure 1.4 Sites of palliative care provision.

Widening access

Activity 1.1

Make a list of people/patient groups who you have seen receive palliative care nursing

Make a list of other people who you think might have unmet palliative care needs

Why do you think this might happen?

Traditionally, palliative care was only offered to patients with a diagnosis of cancer; thankfully in 1998 the government stipulated that the principles and practice of palliative care should become needs led, integral to NHS practices and available to patients, wherever they are, irrespective of diagnosis (DH, 1998). This belief is echoed in the National Service Frameworks (NSF); for example, it is noted that people with heart failure have a worse quality of life than people with most other common medical conditions. There is marked impairment of psychosocial function and over a third of people with heart failure experience severe and prolonged depressive illness (Lynn *et al.*, 1997, Sharpe and Doughty, 1998 both cited in DH, 2000). It is anticipated that most people dying from a non-malignant disease will require palliative care as opposed to specialist palliative care (O'Connor *et al.*, 2011).

In respect to widening access it is also important to ensure that palliative care is available to groups of people who have traditionally been marginalised in relation to the provision of palliative care. These include older people, those with learning disabilities and people from black and ethnic minorities.

Palliative care for older people

Demographics and an increase in long-term conditions and chronic diseases mean that there is a rise in the age of those requiring palliative care (Gardiner *et al.*, 2011). Older people tend to die from one of a few diseases:

- cancer
- cardiovascular
- cerebrovascular
- chronic lung disease
- dementia.

Advanced care planning is vital for older patients to enable them to express their wishes about the care they do and do not receive as their condition progresses. Many older people express an unfulfilled wish to die in their own homes, as most die in care homes or hospitals and a few die in hospices (Gomes *et al.*, 2011).

It is not clear why access to palliative care should differ according to age, but there seems to be a belief amongst some professionals that older people do not have the same palliative care needs as younger people. There is a persistent association between palliative care and cancer diagnosis and those dying from non-malignant diseases are not referred (Gardiner *et al.*, 2011). Health care professionals need to acknowledge that older people have the same palliative care needs as others and should seek out education about caring for older people with palliative care needs.

Challenges increase when providing care for an older person living with dementia. People living with dementia experience symptoms similar to people living with cancer, and experience them for a longer period (WHO, 2011). People living with dementia do not receive adequate palliative care, either because of problems of confirming prognosis or inadequate professional perception of palliative care needs. Communication is difficult which makes assessment and management of symptoms challenging. Advanced care planning needs are to be initiated early on in the disease process (WHO, 2011). Guidelines for the management of symptoms such as agitation, constipation and pain have been introduced on a small scale with some benefit (Lloyd Williams and Payne, 2002)

People living with learning disabilities

People living with learning disabilities experience a number of health inequalities (Emerson and Baines, 2010).

People with learning disabilities are one of the most socially excluded groups in Britain. With poorer health than the general population, they face specific challenges when trying to access end of life care. While people with learning disabilities have more similarities to the rest of the population rather than differences, they cannot access services as easily. Problems of access include challenges of

- lack of awareness of the need for palliative care for the person or their carer;
- lack of confidence of palliative care providers to work with people having learning disabilities;
- informed consent;
- communication – good communication is the key to effective end of life care, yet 50%+ of people with learning disabilities have communication impairment;
- interpretation of behaviour;
- uncertainty of how to raise sensitive issues with people having learning disabilities.

Read and Morris (2008)

Clear communication with family, friends and familiar carers is the key in order to gain information about the person. Carers need to be made aware of when illness or deterioration might be suspected and advised to contact their GP if concerned. Health care professionals need to work at developing creative ways of communicating openly and honestly with people with learning disabilities so that they understand as much as possible and are empowered to make informed choices. This can be achieved by working with the family or familiar carers. Consent, mental capacity and the person's best interests need to be assessed.

Black and ethnic minorities

There is an acknowledged need to extend racially and culturally sensitive palliative care services to the minority ethnic communities, who, because of a lower incidence of most cancers, have historically been unfamiliar with palliative care services. Professional perceptions of how the minority ethnic families respond to life-limiting illnesses have compounded underuse of palliative care service. There is a belief that families care for their own relatives. Whilst the incidence of cancer may be lower in the minority ethnic groups there are a number of life-limiting diseases such as heart and cardiovascular diseases experienced by these groups. There is a clear need for palliative and specialist palliative care (Gunaratnam, 2007). In order to promote equity of timely access to appropriate services, care for these groups should mirror that of the other groups and be informed by the same frameworks and pathways. It is important to promote sensitive responsive services, through working with relevant bodies (Gunaratnam, 2006).

The changes in the focus and provision of palliative care have partly been influenced by government reports and related strategies. These have shaped the development of services since the early days.

Influential documents and strategies

The first attempt to rationalise and coordinate cancer services was through the Calman Hine report (Expert advisory group, 1995) in which it was recognized that palliative care needed to be integrated with other aspects of cancer care. It raised the difference between generalist and specialist palliative care, identifying that both were equally important. These recommendations were adapted by each of the four nations to meet a more local need, for example, the Cameron report (Welsh Office, 1996).

The focus on cancer care has been perpetuated by the NICE guidelines for supportive care (2004) but aspects of these have been adapted to fit non-malignant conditions (NCPC, 2010).

Gold Standards Framework (GSF)

This framework was introduced in 2000 to enable primary care practitioners to improve the supportive and palliative care offered to patients with any end stage illness (Thomas, 2003). It is a systematic evidence-based approach to optimising the care delivered by general health care practitioners to patients nearing the end of their lives. The framework is now used by many practitioners to improve the quality and co-ordination of care provided in a number of settings and aims to enable people to die comfortably in the place of their choice. The GSF has been introduced to a number of different settings including care homes, acute hospitals, community hospitals and prisons and is supported by a comprehensive programme of education, resources and audit. The framework has continued to develop around the seven C's of the community GSF which are the key tasks of patient care (Figure 1.5)

End of life care pathways

The first end of life care pathway introduced was the Liverpool Care Pathway (LCP) which was introduced in England to ensure the delivery of appropriate, evidence-based holistic care for hospital patients in the last days of life. This pathway was also adopted in Scotland and Northern Ireland. Wales developed its own pathway – the All Wales Integrated Care Priorities for the Last Days of Life.

The LCP was developed to facilitate optimal care to dying patients, who were not being cared for in a hospice. It initially focussed on care in the acute sector and was then rolled out into all care settings. In many cases use of the LCP approach to end of life care ensured that patients received appropriate treatment and had a dignified, peaceful death. Unfortunately over the past few years it would appear that implementation of the LCP has not always been appropriate or

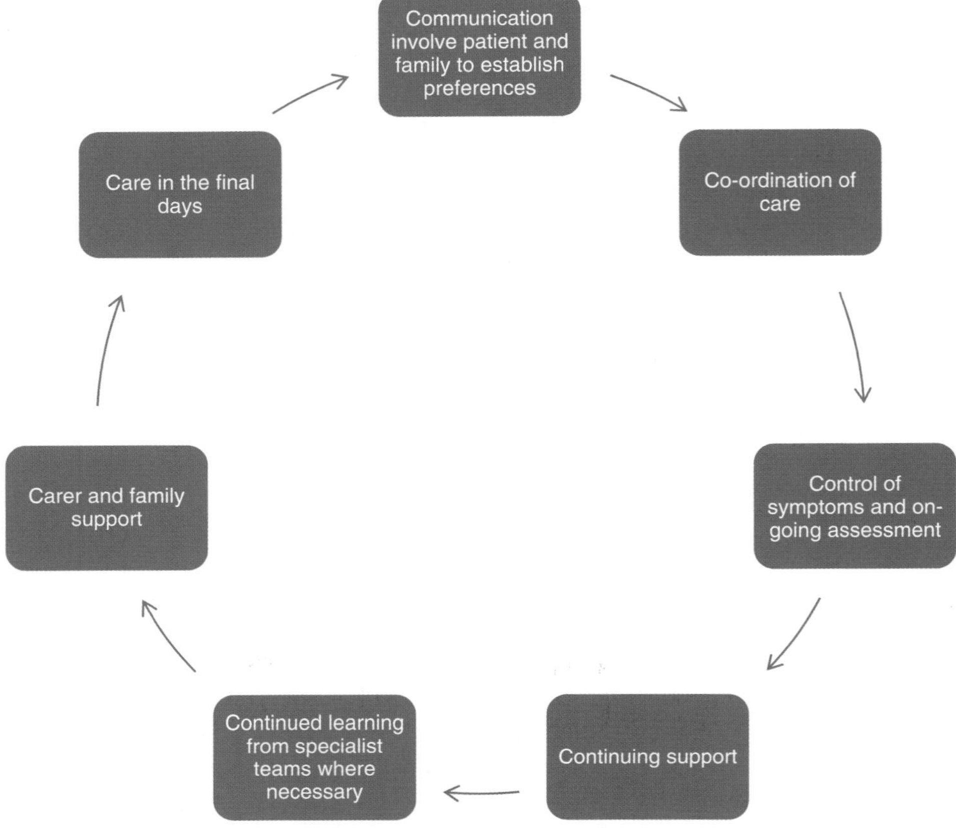

Figure 1.5 The key tasks of patient care (GSF, 2012).

correct because of practitioners' lack of understanding of the approach to care, poor communication skills and lack of knowledge about end of life care. Increasing concerns from media, carers, relatives and professionals over the past couple of years led to a review of the use and experience of the LCP in England.

Concerns highlighted in the review related to perceptions around

- premature/inappropriate withdrawal of nutrition and hydration;
- hastening of death through excessive use of opiates or sedation;
- poor communication about patient's deterioration and prognosis;
- lack of professional compassion, respect, care and knowledge.

The review panel reviewed verbal and oral evidence of care relating to use of the LCP (Department of Health, 2013) and made 44 recommendations. The review found great disparity in the quality of care provided to patients in the LCP:

> It would seem that when the LCP is operated by well trained, well-resourced and sensitive clinical teams, it works well.

> Where care is already poor, the LCP is sometimes used as a tick box exercise, and good care of the dying patient and their relatives or carers may be absent.
>
> *DH (2013: p. 3)*

The overarching recommendation was that:

> Use of the Liverpool Care Pathway should be replaced over the next 6–12 months by an end of life care plan for each patient, backed up by condition-specific good practice guidance.
>
> *DH (2013, p. 10)*

This recommendation was underpinned by others, advocating that

- senior clinicians are involved in any clinical decision making and in discussing end of life decisions with relatives and carers, and documenting that discussion;
- all professionals receive education, training and professional development in end of life care;
- The Nursing and Midwifery Council issues guidance for nurses on good practice in decision making in end of life care;
- named nurses and doctors take responsibility for patient care.

Whilst these recommendations currently apply only to England, it is likely that Scotland and Northern Ireland will review their use of the LCP. Guidance has been issued to guide practice during the re-organisation of end of life care (NCPC, 2013). While the LCP will be phased out it is important that the key principles of end of life care advocated by the end of life care strategy are incorporated in the care plans for patients.

End of Life Care Strategy

This strategy was launched in 2008 with the aim of increasing accessibility to high quality care for all people approaching the end of their life. The strategy, which currently only relates to care in England, is informed by key initiatives such as GSF, advanced care planning and preferred priorities of care. The central tenets are enhanced choice, quality, equality and value for money informed by 10 objectives (DH, 2008):

- increased public awareness and discussion of death and dying;
- people to be treated with dignity and respect at the end of their lives;
- to ensure pain and suffering are minimised and optimal quality of life maintained;
- all people to have access to physical, psychological, social and spiritual care;
- individual needs, priorities and preferences for end of life care to be identified, documented, reviewed, respected and acted upon wherever possible;
- services well coordinated to ensure seamless service;
- high quality care to be provided in the last days of life and following death, in all settings;
- carers to be supported during a patient's illness and after their death;
- health and social care professionals receive the necessary education and training to enable them to provide high quality care;
- services to provide good value for money for the tax payer.

Conclusion

Since the time St Christopher's hospice was opened by Cicely Saunders palliative care has never stopped developing. A number of key policies have shaped the growth and direction of services. There are a number of voluntary and charitable organisations committed to the provision of the best quality palliative care. Supportive and palliative care can be provided in any care setting by well educated health care professionals providing good fundamental care. Specialist palliative care teams may become involved to help care for patients who are faced by complex situations or experiencing symptoms which are particularly hard to resolve. Supportive and palliative care is no longer restricted to patients living with cancer, care must be available according to need, not diagnosis and clear strategies need to be introduced in order to guarantee equity of access for traditionally marginalised groups.

Glossary

Advanced care planning	Documented discussions between patients and professionals to enable patients to express their preferences for their care in the final months of life.
End of life care	Care that helps all those with advanced, progressive and incurable illness to live as well as possible until they die.
Palliative care	The active, holistic care of patients with advanced progressive illness in order to achieve best possible quality of life for patients and their families.
Specialist palliative care	Specialist care provided to a minority of people with complex needs.
Specialist palliative care team	Teams with palliative care as their core speciality, with high level of professional skills and a high staff patient ratio.

References

Department of Health (1998) *Health Service Circular-Palliative Care*. London: DH.

Department of Health (2000) *National Service Framework for Coronary Heart Disease*. Available at http://www.dh.gov.uk/prod_consum_dh/groups/dh_digitalassets/@dh/@en/documents/digitalasset/dh_4057525.pdf [accessed 17 February 2014].

Department of Health (2008) *End of Life Care Strategy; Promoting high quality care for all adults at the end of life* Available at http://www.dh.gov.uk/prod_consum_dh/groups/dh_digitalassets/@dh/@en/documents/digitalasset/dh_086345.pdf [accessed 17 February 2014].

Department of Health (2013) *More Care, Less Pathway: A Review of the Liverpool Care Pathway* Available at https://www.gov.uk/government/uploads/system/uploads/attachment_data/file/212450/Liverpool_Care_Pathway.pdf [accessed 17 February 2014].

Dying Matters (2012) *What is Palliative Care?* Available at http://www.dyingmatters.org/page/what-palliative-care [accessed 17 February 2014].

Emerson, E. and Baines, S. (2010) *Health Inequalities and People with Learning Disabilities in the UK* Available at http://www.improvinghealthandlives.org.uk/uploads/doc/vid_7479_IHaL2010-3HealthInequality2010.pdf [accessed 17 February 2014].

Expert Advisory Group (1995). *A Policy Framework for Commissioning Cancer Services*. London: Department of Health.

Gardiner, C., Cobb, M., Gott, M. and Ingleton, C. (2011) Barriers to providing palliative care for older people on acute hospitals. *Age and Ageing*. 40: 233–238.

Gold Standards Framework (2012) Available at: http://www.goldstandardsframework.org.uk/ [accessed 17 February 2014].

Gomes, B., Calanzani, N. and Higginson, I.J. (2011) *Local Preferences and Place of Death in Regions Within England* Available at http://www.endoflifecare-intelligence.org.uk/resources/publications/lp_and_place_of_death.aspx [accessed 17 February 2014].

Gunaratnam, Y. (2006) *Widening Access to Hospice Care: A Briefing Paper for Managers and Trustees*. London: Help the Hospices.

Gunaratnam, Y. (2007) *Improving the Quality of Palliative Care*. London: Race Equality Foundation.

Lloyd Williams, M., Payne, S. (2002) Can multidisciplinary guidelines improve the palliation of symptoms in the terminal phase of dementia. *International Journal of Palliative Nursing*. 8: 370–375.

National Council for Hospice and Specialist Palliative Care Services (1995) *Specialist Palliative Care: A Statement of Definitions*. London: NCHSPCS.

National Council for Hospice and Specialist Palliative Care Services (1997) *Dilemmas and Directions: The Future of Specialist Palliative Care. A Discussion Paper*. London: NCHSPCS.

National Council for Palliative Care (2010) *Palliative Care Explained* Available at http://www.ncpc.org.uk/palliative_care.html [accessed 17 February 2014].

National Council for Palliative Care (2013) *Guidance for Doctors and Nurses Caring for People in the Last Days of Life* Available at http://www.ncpc.org.uk/publication/guidance-doctors-and-nurses-caring-people-last-days-life [accessed 17 February 2014].

National Institute for Clinical Excellence (2004) *Improving Supportive and Palliative Care for Adults with Cancer*. London: NICE.

O'Connor, M., Harris, R. and Lee, S. (2011) Non-malignant disease: a pathway for quality care at the end of life. *British Journal of Neuroscience Nursing*. 7(2): 470–474.

Read, S., Morris, H. (2008) *Living and Dying with Dignity: The Best Practice Guide to End of Life Care for People with a Learning Disability* Available at http://www.mencap.org.uk/sites/default/files/documents/2009-04/best_practice_guide.pdf [accessed 17 February 2014].

Thomas, K. (2003) *Caring for the Dying at Home: Companions on the Way*. Oxford: Radcliffe Medical Press.

Welsh Office (1996), *Cancer Services in Wales: A Report by the Cancer Services Expert Group*, (*The Cameron Report*), Cardiff: Welsh Office.

World Health Organisation (2011) *Palliative Care for Older People: Better Practice* Available at http://www.euro.who.int/__data/assets/pdf_file/0017/143153/e95052.pdf [accessed 17 February 2014].

WHO (2014) *WHO Definition of Palliative Care* Available at http://www.who.int/cancer/palliative/definition/en/ [accessed 17 February 2014].

2

Holistic care in palliative care

Introduction

Holism and holistic care are fundamental principles of palliative care. The World Health Organisation's (2014) definition of palliative care in Box 2.1 highlights the need for holistic assessment and care in order to attend to all problems that patients might experience during their illness. The chapter explores the concept of total pain,before discussing holism, holistic care and assessment. This is followed by an exploration of spirituality and the importance of spiritual care within palliative care. A brief discussion of the QoL is offered before the conclusion.

Learning outcomes

By the end of this chapter you should be able to

- understand the concept of 'total pain';
- discuss the concept of holistic care;
- recognise the importance of holistic assessment;
- recognise the relevance of spirituality in health care;
- understand the complexity of quality of life.

Fundamentals of Palliative Care for Student Nurses, First Edition. Megan Rosser and Helen C. Walsh.

Companion website: www.wiley.com/go/rosser_walsh/fundamentals_of_palliative_care

Box 2.1 Definition of palliative care (WHO, 2014)

Palliative care is an approach that improves the quality of life (QoL) of patients and their families facing the problems associated with life-threatening illness, through the prevention and relief of suffering by means of early identification and impeccable assessment and treatment of pain and other problems, physical, psychosocial and spiritual.

Box 2.2 Total pain

Rather than reducing pain to a mere physiological 'symptom', it must be seen as physical and emotional, biological and cultural, even spiritual and existential

(*Bendelow and Williams, 1995*)

Total pain

Pain can often be one of the most distressing symptoms identified by patients receiving palliative care, it is not, however, a purely physical experience. It also involves other aspects such as personality, mood, behaviour and social relationships (International Association for the Study of Pain, 2009). The concept of 'total pain' was first coined by Dame Cicely Saunders (1978) who suggested that the pain experience encompassed a range of physical, emotional, social and spiritual factors. A definition of total pain is shown in Box 2.2.

Saunders (1978) suggested that 'total pain' is similar to an iceberg with only 10% visible above the surface. By this she means that the physical manifestations of pain we observe in a patient constitute only a tiny proportion of the total pain he or she is experiencing. While pathophysiological reasons can explain the causes of physical pain, less obvious influences of psychological, spiritual or social factors can exacerbate the patient's experience of pain. Indeed these factors may impact the pain experience more than the disease.

Components of total pain include the following:

- physical pain which arises from the disease, co-morbidities and treatment;
- social pain which results from the impact of the disease on the role and staus of the individual, their financial security and family functioning;
- psychological pain which relates to fear, anxiety and depression;
- spiritual pain which is concerned with existential questions, the search for meaning. For some people spiritual pain also relates to their faith.

Physical pain cannot be treated in isolation; unless all areas are attended to, the patient's pain will persist, even when all appropriate analgesics have been prescribed. Thus an holistic assessment is paramount to the management of total pain.

Holism

Activity 2.1

What does the term holistic care mean to you?

The word holism has its origins in two Greek words, both of which mean 'whole'. This first 'holos', is the stem for holism and the second 'hale' is the stem for healing and health. Health is generally considered to be concerned with the state of a person's mind and body, usually meaning free from illness, injury or pain. Healing is the process of restoring health to a diseased, injured or damaged individual. Mariano (2005) defines healing as the integration of the totality of humankind in body, mind, emotion and spirit—hence its link to holism.

'Holism' in health care is a philosophy that comes directly from Florence Nightingale who encouraged care that focussed on unity, wellness and the interrelationship among human beings, events and the environment (Mariano, 2005). She recognised the importance of such factors as the environment, touch, light, scents, music and silent reflection in the therapy process (Papathanasiou *et al.*, 2013), thus reaching out to patients in ways that went beyond providing only physical care. McEvoy and Duffy (2008) identify four components of holism which are shown below in Box 2.3.

In addition to the components identified by McEvoy and Duffy (2008), Mariano (2005) adds that holism acknowledges and values the inherent goodness of the individual. While individuals have the ability to find meaning and purpose in their lives and experiences, the body also has an innate power to heal itself and it is the nurse's role to support the patient so that they find peace, comfort and harmony (Mariano, 2005).

Holism leads to an holistic approach to care. Holistic care is concerned with the whole, for example, the physical, psychological, social and spiritual aspects of the patient and the family. Papathanasiou *et al.* (2013) identify the holistic approach that

- involves viewing each individual as a separate entity in both biological and social terms;
- is multidimensional and therefore offers a more complex view of health and disease.

With an holistic approach, the person is treated rather than just their symptoms and it is recognised that treatment on one level impacts all other levels (Mariano, 2005). For example, relieving a patient's boredom by offering divisional therapy in a group setting may well meet social and psychological needs which in turn may help relieve pain.

Holistic care

Holistic care is based on a model for care which differs substantially from the traditional biomedical model underpinning Western medicine. These differences are shown in Box 2.4. Within the biomedical model of health care, preserving life is paramount and the focus is on curing the disease or injury. Holistic care however focuses on the individual and what is right for them. The degree of suffering experienced by the patient is more important than the disease and the aim is to heal rather than cure.

Box 2.3 Components of holism (McEvoy and Duffy, 2008)

Holism:

- views the person as a whole;
- is concerned with the interrelationship between body, mind and spirit;
- promotes psychological and physiological well being;
- fosters socio-economic relationships.

Box 2.4 Differences between biomedical and holistic models of care (Cobb and Robshaw, 1998)

Biomedical model	**Holistic model**
Values human life	Values the human being
Focuses on disease/injury	Focuses on suffering
Aims for cure	Aims to heal

Box 2.5 Valerie

Valerie is a 73-year-old lady who was diagnosed with breast cancer several years ago. Following an expected course of treatment, that is, surgery, chemotherapy and radiotherapy, she went on to develop bone and liver metastases. She had been married to Ted for 50 years and was both a mother and grandmother. As her cancer advanced, Valerie experienced increasing physical symptoms and was eventually referred to the specialist palliative care team for symptom control.

Valerie's marriage to Ted had not been happy and as she realised that she was approaching the end of her life, she wanted a divorce. Her words were 'I've been married to the sod for most of my life and I don't want to die married to him'. The specialist team helped with symptom control and supported Valerie in her wish to divorce her husband. This involved considerable work with the family who considered her wish to divorce Ted was 'a bit late in the day' and 'what did it matter now'.

Despite family opposition and increasing weakness as her disease progressed, Valerie continued with her divorce. She received her decree absolute and died peacefully three days later.

The holistic model of care takes into consideration each individual's psychological, sociological and spiritual needs as well as their physical needs (Papathanasiou *et al.*, 2013) and seeks to meet them where they are. Consider Valerie, the patient discussed in Box 2.5.

The specialist palliative care team involved in Valerie's care recognised her need to divorce Ted and facilitated the process. They were able to help with her physical symptoms, but more importantly although they could not cure her, they helped to heal her by enabling her to fulfil her wishes.

Holistic assessment

The Nursing and Midwifery Council (NMC) (2010) expects newly qualified nurses to be able to undertake an holistic person centred assessment. Assessment is the first stage in the nursing process and is an organised, systematic approach to the collection of objective and subjective data about the patient's condition, situation, experiences and disease trajectory. Assessment continues throughout the episode of care and is undertaken through conversation with the patient, observation and examination. Holistic assessment involves asking questions about all aspects of the patient's life in order to gain insight into their physical, psychological, social, emotional and spiritual needs. All information obtained during the assessment is interpreted, analysed and documented by the nurse in order to identify patient problems – both actual and potential.

Activity 2.2

Why do you think holistic assessment is important in palliative care? What do you think are the key nursing skills used in assessment? Jot down your answers and compare them to the lists below.

Holistic assessment is important in palliative care because

- it is the basis of all care;
- it enables nurses to understand the patient's experience and their perceptions of the illness and associated problems;
- it leads to the identification of patients' problems and informs clinical decision making;
- it makes health care professionals aware of the patient's needs and problems;
- it enables patient needs to be prioritised;
- problems and needs determined at the time of assessment influence the nursing care planned and delivered;
- documentation of findings from assessment can service as communication tools between health care professionals;
- information gained from assessment provides baseline data used for evaluation of interventions.

The key nursing skills used during nursing assessments are

- good questioning skills;
- good listening skills;
- good reflective skills;
- good observational skills;
- ability to establish a rapport;
- ability to demonstrate empathy;
- ability to analyse, document and communicate findings from assessment to care.

To provide co-ordinated care the patient and their family need a full holistic assessment of their needs (Nicol, 2011). PEPSI-COLA (Gold Standards Framework, 2005) is an acronym to help guide an holistic assessment in palliative care, highlighting areas which need to be explored with the patient and the family. The meaning of PEPSICOLA is shown in Box 2.6.

One of the key components of holistic care is making assessments that include planning for the future. Advanced care planning (ACP) is a key component of the End of Life Care Strategy (DoH, 2008). ACP anticipates deterioration and explores what the patient and family want to do when the time comes (Nicol, 2011). The process involves and allows open discussion between the patient, family members and the MDT. The purpose of the discussions are summarised in Box 2.7. These discussions need to be documented, regularly reviewed and communicated to key people (Nicol, 2011).

Box 2.6 PEPSICOLA guide to holistic assessment (Gold standards framework, 2005)

Physical – the assessment of symptoms, pain charts, medication review, stopping non essential medication and treatment

Emotional – knowledge and understanding of condition, emotional reactions of patient and family depression

Personal – cultural background, language, sexuality, spiritual and religious needs

Social – social assessment, benefits, carer assessment, aids, preferred place of care

Information and communication

Control and autonomy – mental capacity, treatment options, preferred place of care, advanced care planning, identify potential conflict between wishes of patient and carer

Out of hours communication – on call teams, carer support, night sitters, medication

Late end of life care – last 2 days

After care of family, informing others members of MDT

Box 2.7 Purposes of ACP discussions (DoH, 2008)

- to identify the person's wishes and concerns;
- to identify the person's values and beliefs;
- to establish their understanding of their condition and likely prognosis;
- to establish their preferences for the type of care they want as part of their future management.

Having discussed holism, holistic care and assessment we will now turn to a key component of that holistic care – spirituality.

Spirituality

Defining spirituality is not easy, it is a complex and multi-faceted concept (Amoah, 2011). Spirituality includes an individual's beliefs, values, identity, a sense of meaning and purpose. For some, spirituality will include religion. Wright and Neuberger (2013) describe the 'very stuff' of spirituality to be concerned with how we see ourselves in the scheme of things, how we relate to other human beings and the wider world and how we find meaning, purpose and connection in life. By its very nature spirituality is often subjective, arbitrary and personal. Some definitions of spirituality are shown below in Box 2.8.

Box 2.8 Definitions of spirituality

Spirituality refers to those beliefs, values and practices that relate to the human search for meaning in life. For some people, spirituality is expressed through adherence to an organised religion, while for others it may relate to their personal identities, relationships with others, secular, ethical values or humanistic philosophies.

(NHS, National End of Life Care programme, 2011: p. 6)

Spirituality is that dimension of a person that is concerned with ultimate ends and values . . .. Spirituality is that which inspires in one the desire to transcend the realm of the material

(O'Brien, 1982)

Spirituality is a way of being and experiencing that comes through awareness of the transcendent dimension and that is characterised by certain identifiable values in regard to self, others, nature, life and whatever one considers to be the Ultimate

(Elkins et al., 1988)

Spiritual Care is person centred care which seeks to help people (re)discover hope, resilience and inner strength in times of illness, injury, transition and loss

(NHS Education for Scotland, 2013).

Spiritual care is usually given in a one-to-one relationship, is completely person centred and makes no assumptions about personal conviction or life orientation

(NHS Scotland, 2002)

Spirituality involves the belief in self and others and this may include a belief in a deity or higher power (RCN, 2011). The RCN (2011) also identifies the following as components of spirituality:

- hope
- strength
- trust
- forgiveness
- love
- relationships
- creativity
- self expression.

The experience of advanced illness is often underpinned by existential beliefs and values relating to the meaning, the human condition and purpose of life (Selman *et al.*, 2011). While many can ignore these existential questions during their lives, approaching death brings them sharply into focus (Amoah, 2011). The very nature of spirituality makes it intensely personal, and as a result, specific issues affecting patients may be hard to recognise, but spiritual distress may be manifested in hopelessness, helplessness, anger and lack of comprehension of what is happening.

Spiritual care

Some may argue that because spirituality is so personal it has no place in health care but returning to the concept of total pain it is clear that spiritual care is an essential component of palliative care (NICE, 2004; NHS, 2011). In 2002 Scotland became the first country in the UK to publish a comprehensive strategy for health care and spirituality (NHS Scotland, 2002). This freed spiritual care from the usual limitations of guidelines for religious care (Wright and Neuberger, 2013).

Activity 2.3

What does spirituality mean to you? Consider how you would define spiritual care? What do you think are the key requirements of spiritual care? Compare your answers with those in Box 2.9.

Box 2.9 Spiritual care and its requirements

Spiritual care recognises and responds to the needs of the human spirit when faced with trauma, ill health or sadness and can include the need

- for meaning
- for self worth
- to express oneself
- for faith support
- for a sensitive listener.

(NHS Education for Scotland, 2009).

Spiritual care is about meeting people at the point of their deepest need (RCN, 2011) and begins with encouraging human contact in a compassionate relationship and then moving in whatever direction is needed (NHS Education for Scotland, 2009).

While spirituality and religion are often used interchangeably (Pike, 2011), spiritual care needs to be based on the premise that spirituality is a much broader concept that just religion. O'Brien (2008: p. 4) defines religion as 'a person's beliefs and behaviours associated with a specific religious tradition or denomination'. Formal religion as a means of expressing underlying spirituality (NICE, 2004) is a useful way of understanding and integrating the two concepts (Hayden, 2011).

Box 2.10 Manifesto for Change (Wright and Neuberger, 2012)

1. Spiritual care is not a luxury or an added extra, but goes to the heart of care. Fundamental to how we see each other and our place in the world, it means never viewing those we care for as 'others'. A part of the proper provision of health care, spirituality is not about proselytising or imposing religious beliefs.
2. Education programmes for nurses must provide an in-depth understanding of what people mean by spirituality, its connection to health and well being and must include ways of delivering spiritual care.
3. Education programmes should be imaginative enabling nurses to relate spiritual care to their own spirituality. These programmes should be part of the process of a lifelong learning.
4. Health care environment should provide patients with access to spiritual support through the ability of those who are providing care to form relationships and nurture spiritual needs.
5. As spirituality has a direct effect on health and well being it is a proper area of study and action for **all** involved in health care. As a patient, everybody on the ward is part of the therapeutic team.
6. Many nurses do not understand what it is to provide spiritual care and all nurses should spend time in areas which deliver good practice, for example, palliative care units.
7. Spiritual care contributes to enhancing the healing environment and all nurses can campaign for improving physical environment.

Spirituality is greater than religious beliefs and practices (RCN, 2011) and it is always helpful to view each individual as a spiritual being irrespective of their belief in a higher power (Hayden, 2011). For those with firm religious beliefs it is important to involve an appropriate religious leader in the patient's spiritual care if the patient wishes.

Wright and Neuberger (2013) firmly believe that spirituality is a core aspect of what it means to be human as well as what it means to be a nurse. They acknowledge that very few nurses fully understand spiritual care and that education is essential. As a consequence, they published a seven point manifesto for spirituality and nursing (Wright and Neuberger, 2012) a summary of which is shown in Box 2.10. From this manifesto we can see that spiritual care is not a luxury or add on in health care. It is a fundamental component of enhancing the healing environment.

Providing spiritual care is not about 'doing to', but all about 'being with' an individual and consequently it is our attitudes, behaviours and personal qualities which are important (RCN, 2011).

Activity 2.4

What attitudes, behaviours and personal qualities do you think are needed to give effective spiritual care? While your answers may be very personal, compare them with those identified by the RCN (2011) in Box 2.11.

Box 2.11 Requirements for effective spiritual care (adapted from RCN, 2011)

We need to be able to

- adopt a caring attitude and disposition, responding to the individual where they are, in a non judgemental way;
- recognise and respond appropriately to individual needs, using effective communication skills especially listening and questioning;
- identify clues that may indicate a spiritual need, for example, is the patient sad, angry, or withdrawn? Do they appear helpless or hopeless? What personal material are with them, for example, photographs, religious books or symbols?
- give time to listen to them and to attend to their individual needs;
- recognise when it is appropriate to refer to another source of support, for example, chaplain, counsellor, another staff member, family or friend;
- recognise when we need more support and be willing to seek it out.

Spiritual care begins with the patient and we need to take our cues from them, observing and listening to what they have to say (Smyth and Allen, 2011). In a study of qualified nurses' experiences of assessing spiritual needs, respondents reported that the cues come from patients' interactions with family and staff, sleep patterns, physical pain and emotional distress (Smyth and Allen, 2011). Being with the patient is perhaps the most important thing we can do, conveying our willingness to stay with them at this difficult time. Box 2.12 contains some questions which you might find useful for approaching issues of spirituality with patients.

While a sensitive listener is one of the spiritual care needs identified by NHS Education for Scotland (2009), we must be careful that we do not try and impose our own beliefs and values or use our position to convert another person (RCN, 2011). Sometimes, however, it may be apparent that the patient is seeking some help to support them with their spiritual beliefs. Before taking any action we should consider the points identified in Box 2.13.

Box 2.12 Useful questions for approaching spirituality (RCN, 2011)

- do you have a way of making sense of the things that are happening to you?
- what sources of support or help do you look to when life is difficult?
- would you like to see someone who can help you?
- would you like help to think through or talk about the impact of this illness?

Box 2.13 Considerations in spiritual care (RCN, 2011)

- who initiated or identified the need for help?
- has consent been given?
- does the action that you are considering comply with your professional and employer's code of conduct?
- is it safe and appropriate?
- could it cause offence?
- do you feel comfortable?
- do you have sufficient knowledge and skills?
- is there appropriate support and supervision for you and the patient?

We must remember that spiritual care is not a specialist activity, nor is it the sole responsibility of the chaplain (RCN, 2011). Patients may also receive considerable emotional benefit from the informal support from relatives, friends, religious groups as well as more formal pastoral care.

Quality of life

Optimal QoL is central to palliative care (NICE, 2004; Amoah, 2011). What do we mean by QoL?

Activity 2.5

What do you understand by the term 'quality of life'?

What impacts your own QoL? What makes it better and what makes it worse?

Now think about someone you have nursed who was receiving palliative care.

What do you think their QoL was?

Could you have done anything to improve it?

Compare your answers to the points raised in Box 2.14 and Box 2.15.

Box 2.14 Definitions of quality of life

"a descriptive term that refers to people's emotional, social and physical wellbeing, and their ability to function in the ordinary tasks of living" (Donald, 2003: p. 1)

"a concept representing individual responses to the physical, mental and social effects of illness on daily living which influence the extent to which personal satisfaction with life circumstances can be achieved" (Bowling, 1997: p. 6)

Box 2.15 Factors influencing quality of life (adapted from Wilhelmson *et al.*, 2005; Faithfull, 2003)

- physical functioning and symptoms;
- social and emotional functioning and well being;
- cognitive functioning;
- sexual functioning;
- levels and perceptions of health;
- meaning of the illness to the individual;
- satisfaction with life;
- levels of energy and vitality;
- cultural beliefs;
- economic status.

Maintaining the patient's QoL is, without doubt, a key component of palliative care. It is, however, difficult to define as it is multi-dimensional, dynamic and subjective (Jocham *et al.*, 2006). Kassa and Loge (2003) identify that there is a general agreement that QoL relates to symptom control, physical functioning, psychological and social wellbeing and to a lesser extent meaning and fulfilment. Box 2.14 shows two generic definitions of QoL.

QoL is subjective, multi-dimensional and dynamic. It is also dependent on the individualised context and may vary at different stages of a person's life. For example, walking with a stick or Zimmer frame might be perceived as having a negative effect on the QoL at 18, but at 80 it might make the difference between staying in one's own home or going into a nursing home. Subjective perception of QoL is the key and encompasses the individual's ability to cope, their expectations, levels of optimism and sense of self (Wilhelmson *et al.*, 2005).

At a basic level, assessing the individual's QoL is important as it helps us to plan and evaluate the patient's palliative care. Increasingly, QoL is becoming an important outcome measure in health research, including drug trials. Measuring helps analyse the impact of the disease and treatment upon a person's QoL from an holistic perspective. A formal assessment of the patient's QoL can also be used to make decisions about treatment and to identify the need for focused support (Donald 2003, Corner 2001).

Holmes (2005) has rightly identified that practitioners may know what is right for the patient's disease/illness, but only the patient knows what is best for them, therefore patient centred care must be given in order to optimise patient QoL. Patients may choose to refuse treatment because it reduces their QoL; informed choice is extremely important for patients receiving palliative care. Fallowfield (1990) highlights an interesting dilemma by asking whether the length or quality of survival is most important. Only by delivering sound holistic care may we be able to answer that question.

Conclusion

Holistic care is an important component of palliative care. Recognising that the individual is more than a biophysical being and that the psychological, social and spiritual components are as important allows us to truly give individualised care. Acknowledging the concept of 'total pain' enables us to consider the impact that these other components have on pain and other symptoms. Holistic assessments must be undertaken in order to establish the most effective method of helping the patient, be that pharmacology, creative or complimentary therapies.

Glossary

Advanced illness	A disease which has progressed towards its final stages.
Advanced care planning	Anticipating deterioration and planning care in advance.
Biomedical model of care	A framework for care which prioritises human life, illness/disease and cure.
Deity	A supernatural being who may be thought of as holy, divine or sacred.
Emotional needs	Needs related to feelings.
Ethical beliefs	The beliefs underpinning and contributing to ethical values.
Ethical values	Concerned with right conduct and a good life; actions and behaviours considered good are highly valued while those considered bad are less well regarded.
Existential	Concerned with questions about existence; the 'big' questions of life.
Higher power	A power greater than ourselves.
Holism	Viewing the individual as a whole.
Holistic model of care	A framework that prioritises the individual, suffering and healing.
Holistic care	A multifaceted approach to care encompassing physical, psychological, social and spiritual components.
Humanistic philosophies	A group of beliefs which emphasises the value of human beings.
Multi-dimensional	Something made up of many different components.
Non- judgmental	An approach that accepts the individual and does not form value based opinions.
Nursing process	A framework for organising nursing care, consisting of assessment, planning, implementation and evaluation.

Person centred care	Care which places the individual at its centre.
Physical needs	Relating to needs of the body.
Quality of life	A multi-dimensional subjective concept denoting a person's satisfaction with life.
Religion	An organised formal collection of beliefs, cultural systems and word views that relate humanity to the supernatural.
Religious practices	Those behaviours and rituals whereby a religion expresses its beliefs.
Secular	The state of being separate from religion; worldly.
Self worth	A judgement of and an attitude towards the self.
Spirituality	Relating to those beliefs, values and practices that relate to the human search for meaning.
Spiritual care	Encouraging human contact in a compassionate relationship and meeting people at the point of their deepest need.

References

Amoah, C.F. (2011) The central importance of spirituality in palliative care. *International Journal of Palliative Nursing*. 17 (7): 353–358.

Bendelow, G.A. and Williams, S.J. (1995) Transcending the dualisms; towards a sociology of pain. *Sociology of Health and Illness*. 17 (2): 139–165.

Bowling, A. (1997) *Measuring Health: A Review of Quality of Life Measurement Scales* 2nd edn. Buckingham: Open University Press.

Cobb, M. and Robshaw, V. (1998) *The Spiritual Challenge of Health Care*. Edinburgh: Churchill Livingstone.

Corner, J. (2001) Research and cancer care. In Corner, J. and Bailey, C. (eds) *Cancer Nursing: Care in Context*. Oxford: Blackwell Science, pp. 550–565.

DoH (2008) *Advanced Care Planning A Guide for health and Social Care Staff* 7793 London: DoH.

Donald, A. (2003) *What is Quality of Life?* Available at www.evidence-basedmedicine.co.uk/ebmfiles/whatisQoL.pdf [accessed 17 February 2014].

Elkins, D.N., Hedstrom, L.J., Hughes, L.L., Leaf, J.A. and Saunders, C. (1988) Towards a humanistic-phenomenological spirituality. *Journal of Humanist Psychology*. 28 (4): 5–18.

Faithfull, S. (2003) Assessing the impact of radiotherapy in Faithfull, S., Wells, M. (eds) *Supportive Care in Radiotherapy*. Edinburgh: Churchill Livingstone.

Fallowfield, L. (1990) *The Quality of Life: The Missing Measurement in Health Care*. London: Souvenir Books.

Gold Standards Framework (2005) *PEPSI-COLA Aide Memoir. Palliative Care Monthly Check List*. Walsall: National GSF centre.

Hayden, D. (2011) Spirituality in end-of-life care: attending the person on their journey. *British Journal of Community Nursing*. 16 (11): 546–551.

Holmes, S. (2005) Assessing the quality of life-reality or impossible dream? A discussion paper. *International Journal of Nursing Studies*. 42: 493–501.

International Association for the Study of Pain (2009) *Against Cancer Pain* Available at http://www.iasp-pain.org/AM/Template.cfm?Section=Global_Year_Against_Cancer_Pain&Template=/CM/HTMLDisplay.cfm&ContentID=8716 [accessed 17 February 2014].

Jocham, H.R., Dassen, T., Widdershoven, G. and Halfens, R. (2006) Quality of Life in palliative care: a literature review. *Journal of Clinical Nursing.* 15 (9): 1188–95.

Kassa, S. and Loge, J.H. (2003) Quality of life in palliative care: principles and practice. *Palliative Medicine.* 17 (1): 11–20.

Mariano, C. (2005) *An Overview of Holistic Nursing National Student Nurses' Association Imprint* February/March 48–51.

McEvoy, L. and Duffy, A. (2008) Holistic practice – a concept analysis. *Nurse Education in Practice.* 8: 412–419.

NHS (2011) *Draft Spiritual Support and Bereavement Quality Markers and Measures for End of Life Care* NHS National End of Life Care programme Available at http://www.endoflifecareforadults.nhs.uk/publications/draft-spiriutal-bereavement-cq-markers [accessed 17February 2014].

NHS Education for Scotland (2009) *Spiritual Care Matters: An Introductory Resource for all NHS Scotland Staff.* Edinburgh: NES.

NHS Education for Scotland (2013) *Spirituality* Available at http://www.nes.scot.nhs.uk/education-and-training/by-discipline/spiritual-care.aspx [accessed 17 February 2014].

NHS Scotland (2002) *Guidelines On Chaplaincy And Spiritual Care in the NHS in Scotland.* Edinburg: NHS Scotland.

NICE (2004) *Guidance on Cancer: Improving Supportive and Palliative Care for Adults with Cancer.* London: Spiritual Support Services NICE Available at http://www.nice.org.uk/nicemedia/pdf/csgspman-ual.pdf [accessed 17 February 2014].

Nicol, J. (2011) *Nursing Adults with Long Term Conditions.* Exeter: learning matters Ltd.

Nursing and Midwifery Council (2010) *Standards for Preregistration Education.* London: Nursing and Midwifery Council.

O'Brien, M.E. (1982) The need for spiritual integrity In Yara, H. and Walsh, M. (eds) *Human Needs and the Nursing Process* Vol. 2 Norwalk, CT: Appleton Century Crofts pp. 82–115.

O'Brien, M.E. (2008) *Spirituality in Nursing: Standing on Holy Ground* Massachusetts: Jones and Bartlett.

Papathanasiou, I., Sklavou, M. and Kourkouta, L. (2013) Holistic nursing care: theories and perspectives. *American Journal of Nursing Science.* 2 (1): 1–5.

Pike, J. (2011) Spirituality in nursing: a systematic review of the literature from 2006–2010. *British Journal of Nursing.* 20 (12): 743–749.

Royal College of Nursing (2011) *Spirituality in Nursing Care: A Pocket Guide.* London: Royal College of Nursing.

Saunders, C.M. (1978) *The Management of Terminal Malignant Disease* 1st edn. London: Edward Arnold.

Smyth, T. and Allen, S. (2011) Nurses' experiences assessing the spirituality of terminally ill patients in acute clinical practice. *International Journal of Palliative Nursing.* 17 (7): 337–343.

Selman, L., Harding, R., Gysels, M., Speck, P. and Higginson, I.J. (2011) The Measurement of Spirituality in Palliative Care and the Content of Tools Validated Cross-Culturally: A systematic Review. *Journal of Pain and Symptom Management.* 41 (4): 728–753.

Wilhelmson, K., Andersson, C., Waern, M. and Allebeck P (2005) Elderly people's perspectives on quality of life. *Ageing and society* 25: 585–600.

WHO (2014) *WHO Definition of Palliative Care* Available at http://www.who.int/cancer/palliative/definition/en/ [accessed 18 February 2014].

Wright, S. and Neuberger, J. (2012) Why Spirituality is Essential for Nurses. *Nursing Standard.* 26(40): 19–21.

Wright, S. and Neuberger, J. (2013) Spiritual Expression. *Nursing Standard.* 27 (41): 16–18.

3

Team working

Introduction

This chapter is going to consider many of the different aspects of team work. It will look at what a team is, what team work is and how that working may be improved or impeded. The role of various professionals within the team providing palliative care will be considered.

Learning outcomes

By the end of this chapter you should be able to

- define team, multi-disciplinary and interprofessional team work;
- identify the key members of the palliative care team;
- consider what makes a team function effectively;
- recognise the challenges to effective team work.

Fundamentals of Palliative Care for Student Nurses, First Edition. Megan Rosser and Helen C. Walsh.

Companion website: www.wiley.com/go/rosser_walsh/fundamentals_of_palliative_care

Activity 3.1

Write down a description of a team.

What is a team?

A team is a group of people, often with different knowledge, skills and personalities, working together towards a common goal. In palliative care the goal of an effective team would be the promotion of the best possible quality of life for the patient and their family.

Team work

There are many terms used to denote teams and these are often used interchangeably. However, it may be worth just clarifying that the prefixes multi and inter have different meanings, multi meaning many and inter meaning between – hence definitions can be seen to differ in respect to the level of collaboration.

> **Multi disciplinary team** People from many different professions may be involved in a patient's care but they often act alone and do not collaborate with others.
>
> **Interprofessional team working** Professionals responsible for the patient's care collaborate effectively with each other to improve the quality of care.
>
> Goodman and Clemow (2010)

Collaborative practice

The key difference between multi disciplinary and interprofessional team working is seen to be the feature of collaboration. Collaborative practice is advocated by the World Health Organisation (WHO) (2010) and described as:

> Collaborative practice happens when multiple health workers from different professional backgrounds work together with patients, families, carers and communities to deliver the highest quality of care
>
> *(WHO, 2010: p. 7).*

Activity 3.2

Write down all the benefits of team work that you can think of and compare your answer to the list below.

Benefits of team work

- enables provision of holistic care for patients;
- higher quality of care with continued improvement of care;
- more responsive services for patients;
- better patient outcomes;
- better utilisation of resources;
- increased cost effectiveness;
- enhanced problem solving;
- enables more satisfying roles and improved morale, reduces staff turnover and absenteeism;
- improves patient understanding;
- increases knowledge of team members as they learn from each other.

Fletcher (2008), Goldsmith *et al.* (2010)

The positive outcomes of team work listed above confirm that team work is central to effective health care. The NMC (2010) stipulates that nurses must

- work cooperatively within teams and respect the skills, expertise and contributions of their colleagues;
- be willing to share their skills and experience for the benefit of their colleagues;
- consult and take advice from colleagues when appropriate;
- treat their colleagues fairly and without discrimination;
- make a referral to another practitioner when it is in the best interests of someone in their care.

Activity 3.3

Think why we might need collaborative, interprofessional team work in palliative care.

Why is interprofessional team work important in palliative care?

Patients and families receiving palliative care often have complex needs which could be physical, psychological, social or financial. Thinking back to the composition of a team – that is, people with different skills and knowledge, it is likely that a team approach to patient problems will result in better problem resolution. Each professional group will view a problem differently and the combinations of different views allow a more comprehensive overview of the situation and generation of possible solutions. It is not really possible to provide good palliative care in isolation from other professionals. The WHO definition of collaborative practice echoes the principles of palliative care in pursuit of 'highest quality of care'.

With growing emphasis on extending palliative care to all those with identified clinical need there will be an increase in the number of professionals involved in palliative care. It is vital that they are willing to learn from each other. Team work is one of the central tenets of the principles of palliative

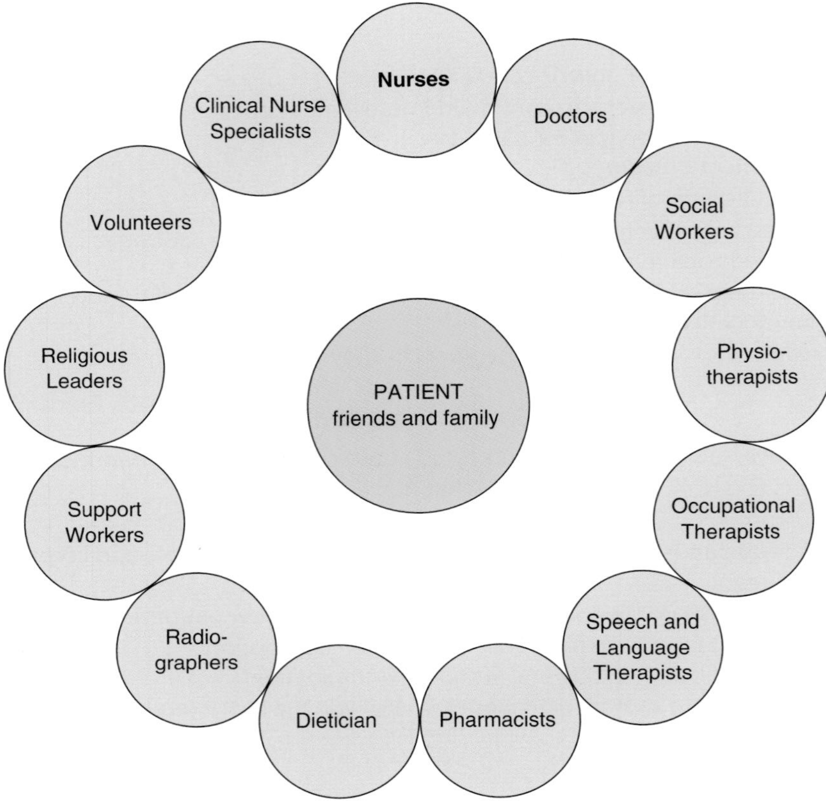

Figure 3.1 Members of the palliative care team.

care, palliative care 'uses a team approach to address the needs of patients and their families' (WHO, 2013). Figure 3.1 shows who the main people involved in providing palliative care are.

Activity 3.4

Having seen who might be in the team, have a go at writing down what their role might be in caring for a patient with palliative care needs, and their family.

Nurses	
Clinical nurse specialists	

Doctors	
Support workers	
Social workers	
Physiotherapists	
Occupational therapists	
Speech and language therapists	
Pharmacists	
Dietician	
Radiographer	
Religious leaders	
Volunteers	

Now compare your answers to the activities listed against each group in Table 3.1:

Table 3.1 The role of professionals involved in the delivery of palliative care.

Nurses	Assessment of patient needs, co-ordination of care Provision and evaluation of nursing care and basic palliative care for patient and family Referring to specialist palliative care team if need identified
Clinical Nurse Specialists	May be specialist in palliative care or chronic conditions Temporary involvement with patient and family to resolve problems – physical, emotional, psychological, financial, spiritual – that the general nurses lack knowledge, time or confidence to deal with Liaison with members of specialist palliative care team as necessary for patient care Education of general healthcare practitioners about aspects of chronic conditions or palliative care
Doctors	Medical assessment of patients Liaison with medical colleagues to ensure patient information is current Responding to basic palliative care needs of patients and their families Prescription of appropriate medications for holistic symptom control Referral to specialist services if need arises
Support Workers	Provision of physical care of patients Possibly provision of basic psychological care for patients and their families (depending on skills set and education) Liaison with nurses in charge of patient care
Social Workers	Advise about benefits, community services and possible residential placements Attention to financial issues – income maintenance, debt counselling Psychological support for patients and families Liaison with social services and other care agencies Advocacy
Physiotherapists	Rehabilitation Attention to physical problems arising from disease or treatment, for example, lymphoedema, breathlessness Promotion of independence and appropriate fitness and exercise regimes Involvement in pain management regimes-through physical therapies, for example, massage, exercise
Occupational Therapists	Rehabilitation Helping patients adapt to change made by the disease or treatment, for example, amputation, hemiplegia Maintenance of quality of life through patient support for engagement with daily living activities which patient finds meaningful

Speech and language therapist	Assessment, diagnosis and care of patients with communication or swallowing difficulties Provision of alternative communication systems
Pharmacists	Promote the rational and optimal use of medication Support and advice for colleagues prescribing medication Patient counselling and education about medication regimes to aid patient concordance
Dietician	Undertaking a nutrition assessment Advising colleagues regards dietary and feeding regimes Teaching patients and families about diet to help them make choices about food and diet supplements
Radiographer	Diagnostic radiographers – diagnosis of disease progression or complication Therapy radiographers – provision of palliative radiotherapy for pain or symptom management
Religious leaders	Pastoral care Contact with local communities Provision of religious rites and practices Advice to staff about acceptable practices for individuals Spiritual and psychological support for patients and families
Volunteers	Support and befriending of patients and families

Most of these groups will work in many of the care settings so team involvement in palliative care is possible in all settings. Whilst some activities, such as radiotherapy, are provided by one professional group many others are not the sole domain of one profession. Practitioners may undertake some of the more general care activities listed above as the role of other professionals. Many of the people listed would be able to provide psychological support for their patients. This can lead to a blurring of professional boundaries and this needs to be managed in order to promote effective team work.

The central activities of any team providing palliative care for patients include

- initial consultation and referral for investigation;
- initial diagnosis;
- review of disease progression;
- communication of diagnosis, disease progression and prognosis to patient, family and relevant health care professionals;
- development and agreement of holistic treatment plans for the patient;
- implementation and evaluation and review of care;
- facilitating advanced care planning;
- support of patient, family and friends throughout.

Patients may receive care from a number of teams, for example, a patient with end stage heart failure may be seen by the cardiac team, the chronic disease management team, the primary health care team and the specialist palliative care team. Teams often consist of core and extended members, core members are involved in the day to day care of the patients and extended members are invited in when the patient situation requires their specialist input (Box 3.1).

Activity 3.5

Read the following patient scenarios and think who might be involved in the patient's care and why.

Patient scenarios

Box 3.1 Patient one

Asha Sidhu is a 54-year-old married lady. Asha was diagnosed with motor neurone disease 2 years ago and retired from her job as a primary teacher 18 months ago when her restricted mobility made it impossible for her to carry on working. Her husband Akal continued to work as a fireman and finds that the shift pattern in his work helps to give him time with Asha. Their son Jai is a policeman and lives about five miles away with his wife and young family, and their daughter Mannat still lives at home and is in her final year of teacher training. Mannat and Akal are managing to provide Asha's personal care between them.

Since diagnosis Asha's mobility has continued to deteriorate, her balance is extremely poor; she experiences joint pain and uses a wheelchair outside the house. Asha has had sacral pressure ulcers in the past but her skin is intact at the moment. Recently Asha has been experiencing increasing difficulty in swallowing; she finds it difficult to chew foods and sometimes chokes when eating or drinking. Asha's speech is also deteriorating.

See Figure 3.2 for members of Asha's palliative care team and Box 3.2 for clarification of their roles (Box 3.3):

Box 3.2 Role of professionals involved in Asha's care

District Nurse (DN) was involved since the incidence of pressure ulcers. Has remained involved and is providing on-going support for Asha and her family. Reviews manual handling assessment and liaises with the physio for advice about transfers and mobility aids.

Also undertakes regular risk assessment for pressure ulcer development and provides pressure relieving aids when necessary.

G.P. visited recently at the request of DN to assess deterioration of speech and swallowing. Considering referral to surgeons for Percutaneous endoscopic gastrostomy (PEG) feeding tube, liaises with SALT to ensure timely referral.

Speech and language therapist (SALT) asked to visit by DN to assess Asha's speech and swallowing. Will liaise with dietician regarding possible thickeners and dietary supplements. Will provide feedback to DN and G.P about the need for a PEG tube. Will provide alternative communication systems for Asha if talking becomes too much of a challenge.

Dietician – asked to advise about dietary supplements and fluid thickeners to maintain nutrition and prevent likelihood of Asha choking as her swallowing reflex gets worse.

Physiotherapist – involved for advice regarding transfer and mobility aids. Provides passive exercises for relief of joint pain – teaches Akal and Mannat how to move and massage Asha's legs to provide relief.

Community pharmacist – chats to Akal and Mannat when they come to collect Asha's medications and also liaises with the GP and DN regarding 'easiest' preparations for administering Asha's medications.

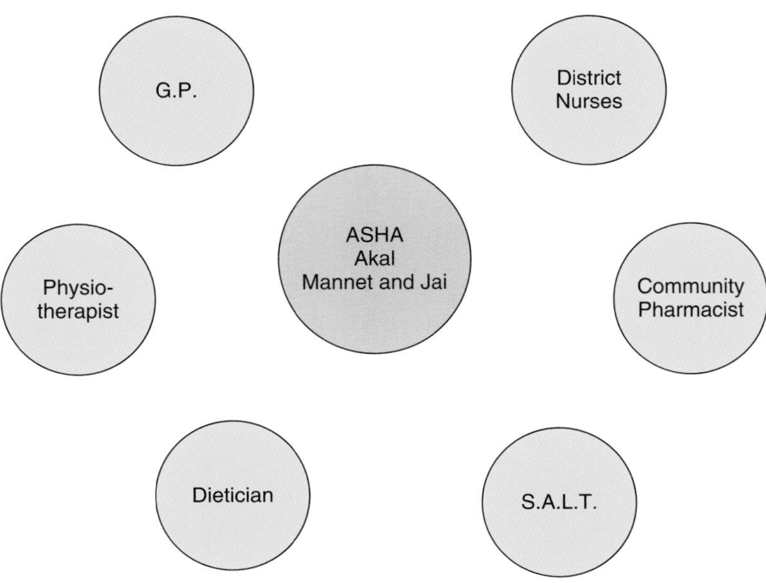

Figure 3.2 Members of Asha's palliative care team.

Box 3.3 Patient two

John Smith is a 65-year-old man; John has had two heart attacks in the past and was diagnosed with heart failure 3 years ago. John lives with his wife Florrie who has rheumatoid arthritis and is finding it increasingly difficult to care for herself, John does a lot of the work at home. They have two grown children who live far away. John and Florrie have been very involved in the local church for years and gain a lot of support from their vicar and friends in the congregation.

John was admitted to a medical ward in his local hospital with an exacerbation of breathlessness, his ankles are oedematous and he is feeling very lethargic. John's appetite is very poor and he has lost a stone in the past three weeks. On examination it is found that he has a chest infection and that his heart failure has progressed. The consultant has explained to John and Florrie that his disease is progressing and that his prognosis is poor-the ward staff have noticed a decline in John's mood since that conversation. John has expressed a strong desire to go home as soon as possible. With winter coming he is worried about how they will keep their home warm.

See Figure 3.3 for the professionals involved in John's care and Box 3.4 for explanations of their roles.

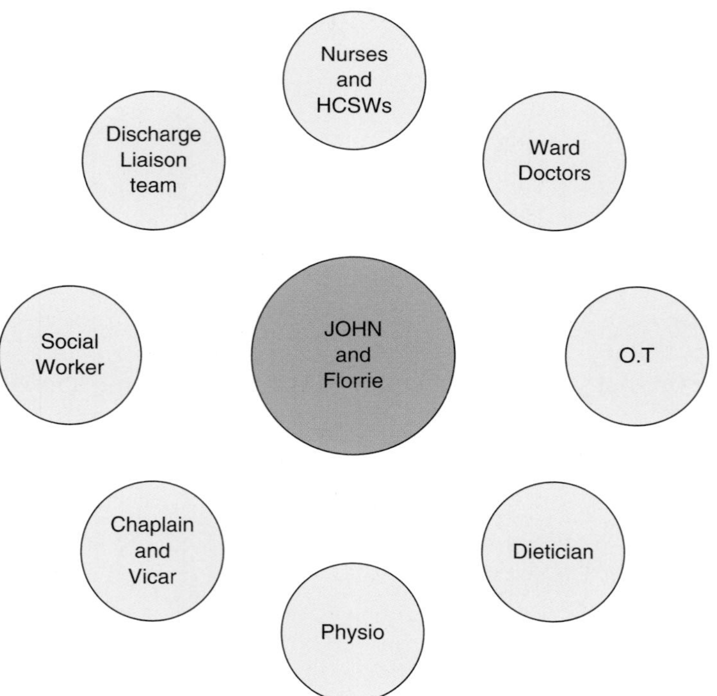

Figure 3.3 Members of John's palliative care team.

Box 3.4 Role of professionals involved in John's care

Ward nurses and health care support workers – assessment of John's needs and provision of holistic nursing care. Referral to other members of the team as and when necessary.

Ward doctors – monitoring of John's physical and emotional condition. Prescription of appropriate medication to alleviate symptoms. May refer to other specialities.

Occupational therapist – assessment of John's capabilities, home visit to assess need for home adaptations in light of John and Florrie's deterioration.

Dietician – nutritional assessment and nutritional advice to prevent further weight loss.

Physiotherapist – for help with acute exacerbation of breathlessness due to infection. Teaching of breathing exercises to help John cope with increasing breathlessness as his heart failure progresses.

Hospital chaplain and local vicar – provision of religious and spiritual care and support for John and Florrie. Vicar will keep members of their local church up to date on John's condition (with John's permission) and may co-ordinate visiting rota and lifts for Florrie if she needs them.

Social worker – to help see if John and Florrie are claiming all they are entitled to.

Discharge liaison team – to ensure all community services are established before John is discharged.

What makes a team work well?

Activity 3.6

Think of a team that you have been part of, that worked well; spend some time thinking why that team worked well and make some notes. (it does not have to be a team at work, it could be any team you have been involved with – for example, a sports team).

Now think of a team that you have been part of that did not work so well – why was that? – jot down your answers (Figure 3.4).

There are classic texts exploring how teams develop and function (Tuckman, 1965; Tuckman and Jensen, 1977; Belbin, 1981) the following sections will consider what facilitates effective team work and what hinders it.

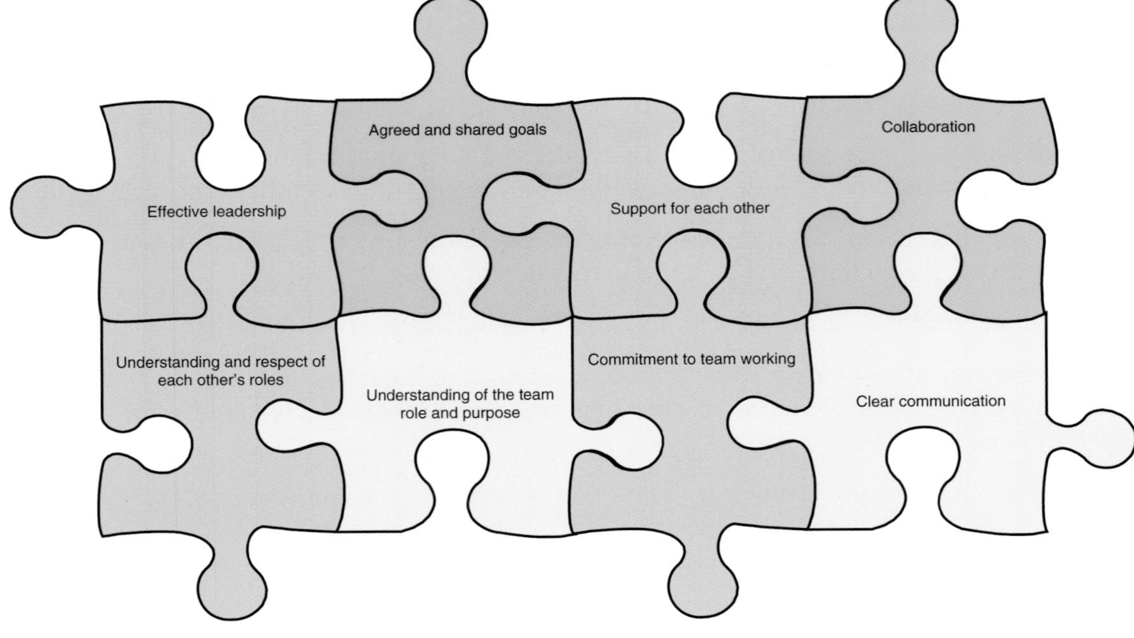

Figure 3.4 What makes a good team?

Agreed and shared goals

A strong team has a common ideal (Spruyt, 2011), in palliative care that will be promotion of the best quality of life for the patient throughout their illness. Smaller goals such as agreeing on the priorities of care would need to be negotiated within the team to ensure co-ordination of care. Failure to clarify goals and team purpose can lead to tension within the team; therefore, it is important to give the whole team time to reach consensus especially in complex or challenging patient situations.

Commitment to team working

For a team to function effectively, members must be committed to the team and believe in its purpose. The team will not work if 'members' only pay lip service to the idea of the team and continue to work in isolation. A team does not evolve because there is a group of people working together, productive team work requires persistent effort to ensure that the team keeps functioning (Sargeant *et al.*, 2008).

Mutual understanding and respect

A strong team must have a shared understanding of the team role and the contributions each individual can make to ensure successful team outcomes (Spruyt, 2011). Mutual professional respect is fostered through a good understanding of each other's roles, and scope of practice (Sargeant *et al.*, 2008). Newer members of the team may have to prove their worth in order to gain respect and true membership of the team (Belanger and Rodriguez, 2008).

Clear effective leadership

A team leader can encourage or discourage collaboration, therefore, it is vital to have an effective, transformational leader. Teams without clear leadership are less effective and more stressful for team members (Fletcher, 2008), conversely strong leadership augments team growth (O'Neil and Cowman, 2008). The most effective leaders demonstrate commitment, effective communication, ability to coach others, flexibility and respect for other's capabilities (Hall *et al.*, 2008).

Leadership can be shared and rotated according to the problem in hand to ensure that the most appropriate professional is leading the team (Hall *et al.*, 2008; McCallin and McCallin, 2009). One of the key tasks of the leader is to ensure that the team has sufficient knowledge to attend to patients needs; therefore, it makes sense that team leadership varies in relation to the patient being cared for. If the patient's main needs relate to rehabilitation either the physio or occupational therapist would be the most appropriate team leader for that episode of care. Conversely if the patient presents with complex physical symptoms it would be appropriate for the doctor to lead the team. Rotation of leadership can enhance integration (Cioffi *et al.*, 2010) and is recommended by NICE (2004).

Communication

Effective communication is vital to establish roles and responsibilities and to foster productive relationships. Open communication enables members to express views, thoughts and feelings without fear. Conflict can be productive if handled sensitively and constructively and honest, sensitive feedback is important to facilitate growth (Goodman and Clemow, 2010). If effective communication is to occur, professionals need both good communication skills and access to team colleagues (Sargeant *et al.*, 2008).

Communication will occur both formally in meetings or telephone conversations and informally through passing comments on the ward or in the surgery. Time has to be dedicated to formal communication within the team. Ward rounds, ward meetings and patient handovers on the ward will facilitate communication within the team, as will practice meetings and case reviews in the community. The specialist palliative care teams will also have regular interprofessional team meetings.

Possession of good interpersonal skills is vital if team members are to communicate with each other. Key interpersonal skills for effective team work include

- active listening skills;
- problem solving;
- decision making;
- verbal and non verbal communication skills;
- assertiveness;
- stress and anger management;
- conflict resolution.

Support for each other

Providing palliative care and end of life care exposes health care professionals to repeated sadness, suffering and ethical dilemmas. This area of care is demanding and potentially exhausting (Pereira *et al.*, 2012). Care and support helps prevent burnout. Appropriate support mechanisms such as reflective practice, clinical supervision, debriefing sessions and clinical audit need to be in place to support the whole team. A supportive team has been noted to be a cornerstone of palliative care as it provides opportunities to share difficult cases and feeling with colleagues (Meier and Beresford, 2008).

What stops a team from working well?

A poorly functioning team can be one of the greatest causes of stress for those involved in providing palliative care and therefore it is important to consider why teams do not always work so well. Obviously issues which impede effective team working are often the exact opposite of the factors facilitating effective team working. There is great potential for teams not to function effectively because they consist of a number of professionals from disparate backgrounds with different agendas (Fletcher, 2008). This disparity within a team may lead to lack of knowledge about each other's roles and consequently lack of professional respect (Sargeant *et al.*, 2008). As stated previously effective intra-team communication helps to overcome these potential problems.

Factors which impede effective team working are shown in Figure 3.5.

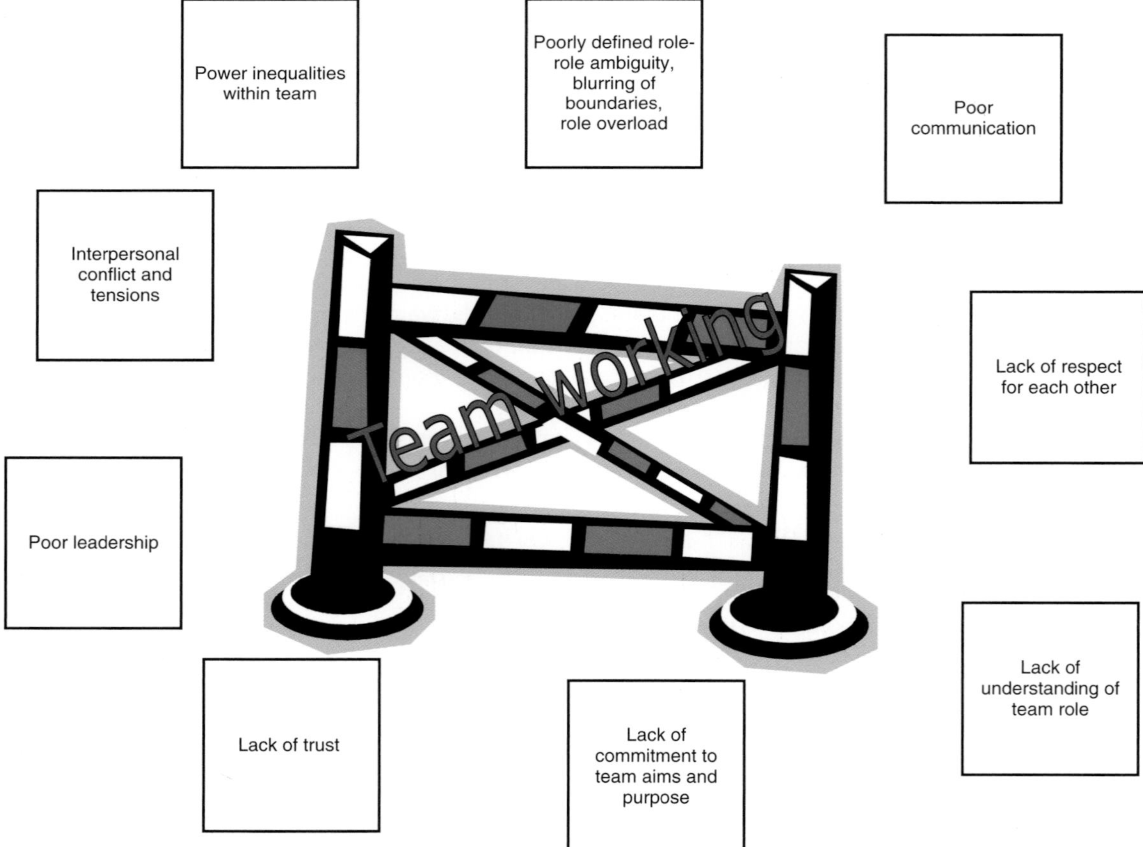

Figure 3.5 What stops a team from working well?

Poorly defined roles and problems with roles

Poorly defined roles and responsibilities within a team can lead to role ambiguity with blurring of boundaries causing confusion. This confusion and lack of clarity causes some team members to feel underutilised whilst others experience role overload. Role ambiguity occurs when a member of the team does not know what is expected of them – this can occur in palliative care because some aspects of care can be given by a number of people. Professionals experiencing prolonged role ambiguities can experience a loss of self confidence, performing less well in their role, consequently there is a lack of team cohesion. Role overload occurs when the work expected from one of the team members far exceeds what he or she is able to do. As that person tries to take on more and more of the patient's care, stress mounts and they cannot do their job well and errors may occur. If roles are not clearly defined there are risks that some jobs will not get done, without clear roles team members may think someone else has done the job.

Interpersonal conflict and tensions

Whilst the outcome of conflict can be constructive most conflicts and tension impacts negatively on a team's ability to perform well. A healthy functioning team deals with conflict more positively. Teams lacking clear and effective leadership are less able to deal constructively with conflicts or tension. Conflicts and tension within a team may arise for a number of reasons, for example:

- roles and responsibilities;
- perceived power imbalances;
- different personal or professional opinions, these could be different opinions about treatment and care options within the team;
- lack of access to other team members for advice about patient care;
- reluctance of some individuals to refer appropriately, preferring to try and provide all care for the patient on their own, working in isolation;
- poor perceptions between professional groups about scope of practice;
- perceived differences in levels of accountability;
- lack of mutual support causing individuals to retreat from team functioning.

Lack of conflict resolution can lead to loss of trust or respect between team members and lack of commitment to the team.

Leadership problems

Teams lacking effective leadership will not perform well and patient care will suffer. Poor leadership can arise because of the personal characteristics of the leader or the leadership style adopted. A poor leader may lack the leadership and interpersonal skills required to gain the team's trust and commitment. Their adopted leadership style may be harsh and rigid, preventing team members from developing as they would under the guidance of a transformational leader.

Inadequate communication

Often different professional groups will blame each other for breakdown in communication, pressure of time is also believed to impede effective communication with each professional group being too busy to take time to communicate. The increased use of technologies in communication in health care creates more opportunities for communication breakdown between team members and many team members still want to rely on verbal relay of important issues (Flicek, 2012). Poor communication within a team can be overcome by use of the SBAR framework– situation, background, assessment and recommendation.

Conclusion

Effective team working promotes holistic patient care and improves patient outcomes. It is, therefore, important in any aspect of health care and vital in palliative care because of the potential complexity of patient and family needs. A number of professions in a variety of teams may be involved in providing palliative care in any health care setting for those who need it. Effective teamwork relies on a clear team purpose, commitment to that purpose with mutual respect and understanding of different roles within the team. Strong, appropriate leadership and optimal supportive communication between members is vital. Teams will not work well if there is a lack of understanding or a lack of appreciation of roles. Poor leadership and inadequate communication also prevent teams from working effectively.

Glossary

Collaborative practice — Members of different professions work together with patients, families, carers and communities to deliver highest possible quality of care.

Interprofessional team — Team comprised of members of different professions who work collaboratively to provide optimal patient care.

Multidisciplinary team — 'Team' comprising of members of different professions who work in isolation from each other to provide their aspect of patient care.

Role ambiguity — Team member uncertain about what their role is within patient care.

Role overload — Team member expected to do far more than they can actually achieve within their role.

SBAR — Framework to guide effective communication between professionals, stating situation, background, assessment and recommendation in any patient situation.

Team — A group of people with different knowledge, skills and personalities working together towards a common goal.

References

Belanger, E. and Rodriguez, C. (2008) More than the sum of its parts? A qualitative research synthesis on multi-disciplinary primary care teams. *Journal of Interprofessional Care.* 22(6): 587–597.

Belbin, R.M. (1981) *Management Teams: Why They Succeed or Fail.* New York: John Wiley & Sons.

Cioffi, J., Wilkes, L., Cummings, J., Wearne, B. and Harrison, K. (2010) Multidisciplinary teams caring for clients with chronic conditions: experiences of community nurses and allied health professionals. *Contemporary Nurse.* 36(1–2): 61–70.

Fletcher, M. (2008) Multi-disciplinary team working: building and using the team. *Practice Nurse.* 35(12): 42–47.

Flicek, C.L. (2012) Communication: a dynamic between nurses and physicians. *Medsurg Nursing.* 21(6): 385–6.

Goldsmith, J., Wittenberg-Lyles, E., Rodriguez, S. and Sanchez-Reilly, S. (2010) Interdisciplinary geriatric and palliative care team narratives: collaboration practices and barriers. *Qualitative Health Research.* 20(1) 93–104.

Goodman, B. and Clemow, R. (2010) *Nursing and Collaborative Practice: A Guide to Interprofessional Learning and Working.* 2nd edn. Exeter: Learning Matters.

Hall, P., Weaver, L., Handfield-Jones, R. and Bouvette, M. (2008) Developing leadership in rural interprofessional palliative care teams. *Journal of Interprofessional Care.* 22(S1): 73–79.

McCallin, A. and McCallin, M. (2009) Factors influencing team working and strategies to facilitate successful collaborative teamwork. *New Zealand Journal of Physiotherapy.* 37(2): 61–67.

Meier, D.E. and Beresford, L. (2008). The palliative care team. *Journal of Palliative Medicine.* 11(5): 677–81.

NICE (2004) *Supportive and palliative care: Improving supportive and palliative care for adults with cancer.* London: NICE.

NMC (2010) *The Code: Standards of Conduct, Performance and Ethics for Nurses and Midwives.* London: NMC.

O'Neill, M., Cowman, S. (2008) Partners in care: investigating community nurses' understanding of an interdisciplinary team-based approach to primary care. *Journal of Clinical Nursing.* 17: 3004–3011.

Pereira, S.M., Fonesca, A.M., Carvalho, A.S. (2012) Burnout in nurses working in Portuguese palliative care teams: a mixed methods study. *International Journal of Palliative Nursing.* 18(8): 373–381.

Sargeant, J., Loney, E., Murphy, G. (2008) Effective interprofessional teams: 'contact is not enough' to build a team. *Journal of Continuing Education in the Health Professions* 28(4): 228–234.

Spruyt, O. (2011) Team networking in palliative care. *Indian Journal of Palliative Care.* 17: S17–S19.

Tuckman, B.W. (1965) Developmental sequence in small groups. *Psychological Bulletin.* 63: 384–399.

Tuckman, B.W. and Jensen, M.A.C.. (1977). Stages of small group development revisited. *Group and Organizational Studies.* 2: 419–427.

World Health Organisation (2010). *Interprofessional Education and Collaborative Practice. Technical Report.* Geneva, Switzerland: World Health Organisation.

WHO (2013) *WHO Definition of Palliative Care* Available at http://www.who.int/cancer/palliative/definition/en/ [accessed 15 February 2014].

4

Legal principles in palliative care

Chantal Patel

Introduction

Nursing practice is underpinned by law. It is imperative to provide palliative care in accordance with the legal and professional obligations as dictated by the state. Ignorance of the law is no defence and, therefore, you cannot provide care in ignorance of the law. As a result of the recent controversy around the Liverpool care pathway (LCP), the Francis report as well as the Keogh report, it is now more important than ever to be able to justify the provision of care to patients with palliative care needs. The Nursing Midwifery Council provides the relevant guidance for safe and effective practice safely. In contrast, the law delineates what you are permitted to do.

Learning outcomes

At the end of the chapter you will be able to

- identify the pertinent legal issues in relation to care and treatment at end of life;
- discuss the law in relation to life-sustaining treatment;
- outline issues associated with euthanasia;
- understand the process of deciding not to resuscitate;

Fundamentals of Palliative Care for Student Nurses, First Edition. Megan Rosser and Helen C. Walsh.

Companion website: www.wiley.com/go/rosser_walsh/fundamentals_of_palliative_care

- understand the difference between withholding and withdrawing treatment;
- explain the requirements for verification of expected death.

Activity 4.1

Consider whether you have total freedom to make the following decisions:

	Dictated by your own professional duties	Dictated by the law
1. Withdraw care and treatment		
2. Share patient information		
3. Withhold information from patient		
4. Sedate		
5. Do not resuscitate		
6. Administer blood transfusion		

In doing so, you will have noticed that some of these decisions are guided by both professional and legal duties. None of these actions can be carried out without cognizance of the law. In short, whatever we do for the patient will be underpinned by both professional and legal obligations. As a nurse you will find that the law is based on general principles, which need to be applied to the relevant context. Consequently, the nurse needs to have an understanding of these general legal principles as applicable to palliative care. The nature of palliative care entails a discussion around issues focusing on end of life, what can be done to support the patient in a dignified manner while respecting the wishes of the patient pre- and post-death.

Identification of legal issues surrounding the provision of palliative care

Healthcare professionals are often under public scrutiny for the ethical and legal dilemmas they face in end of life care. The concerns around poor care, in particular of the elderly as well as those perceived to have a poor quality of life are highlighted in the Francis report and the review of the LCP. In a nutshell, the main issues centre on

- approaches to decision-making at the end of life;
- the role of consent;
- withholding and withdrawing of treatment;
- assisted nutrition and hydration;
- cardiopulmonary resuscitation;

- the validity of an advance directive;
- the role of the lasting power of attorney (LPA);
- the role of the independent mental capacity advocate;
- the use of opiates to control pain;
- the donation of organs post-death (Box 4.1).

Consent

The law provides that adults have a right to determine what happens to their bodies. In Schloendorff v Society of New York hospitals (1914) "Every human being of adult years and sound mind has a right to determine what shall be done with his own body; and a surgeon who performs an operation without his patient's consent commits an assault for which he is liable in damages. This is true except in cases of emergency where the patient is unconscious and where it is necessary to operate before consent can be obtained". While this is an American case, it captures the essence of consent. It is noted that this case is of persuasive value within the jurisdiction of the United Kingdom. It is, therefore, essential that nurses seek appropriate permission from the

Box 4.1 Case study: snapshot of the findings of the review of the Liverpool care pathway

The LCP came about as a result of successful models of care developed in hospices. The LCP is a generic model to manage the care of the dying. Concerns were raised by relatives of the poor and the undignified care received by their loved ones in the days leading to their death. One article in the Daily mail of 15 July 2013, reported that *Dying patients were placed on the LCP without their families knowing, left for weeks and in some cases months, and denied water despite the pleading of loved ones to let them have a drink.*

The review uncovered similar issues of poor care raised at Mid Staffs. Here is a summary of the key issues in the review:

- poor documentation;
- poor communication between relatives and staff about the clinical condition of the patient;
- decision making often made in the middle of the night, at weekends or bank holidays without consultation with a senior responsible clinician;
- confusion around consent;
- lack of involvement of carers in the care plan;
- lack of understanding around assisted hydration and nutrition;
- inappropriate use of sedation;
- do not resuscitate was implied by clinical staff as a proxy for agreement to start the LCP;
- lack of understanding between relieving pain and hastening death;
- unclear who is accountable for decisions taken;
- poor care of the elderly.

The Liverpool Review demonstrates that an understanding of the law in relation to consent, withdrawal of treatment and record keeping is an essential aspect of palliative care.

Box 4.2 Case Study: RE MB (Caesarean section [1997] CA)

Baroness Elizabeth Butler-Sloss stated 'The right to determine what shall be done with one's body is a fundamental right in our society. The concepts inherent in this right are the bedrock upon which the principles of self-determination and individual autonomy are based. Free individual choice in matters affecting this right should, in my opinion, be accorded very high priority'.

patient to provide any care. Liability for failure to do so can be either a claim of trespass to the person, that is, the person did not agree to the treatment given; or negligence where the patient was not given the relevant material information upon which agreement can be based. Further, there is recognition that capacity can fluctuate from decision to decision, and therefore, consent obtained is decision specific (Box 4.2).

The statement made by Baroness Butler-Sloss demonstrates the importance of seeking agreement from the patient prior to any interventions. However, this seemingly inalienable right is predicated on the capacity of the patient, that is, the patient needs to demonstrate that he or she has an understanding of the nature of the treatment that is being proposed including any consequences that may ensue, should they refuse.

For consent to be valid the patient needs to

- be given information that is materially relevant that enables the patient to make a decision;
- understand the nature of the treatment proposed including any side effects as well as the potential of death, should they decline any treatment offered;
- have arrived at this decision without being influenced or coerced into making this decision;
- be able to communicate this decision to the treating team.

Activity 4.2

Understanding capacity: consider the scenarios below

1. A 52-year-old lady, with limited ability to communicate because of motor neurone disease, and who can only communicate with a very tiny movement of one eyelid, informs her carers and her medical team that if her heart stopped she would not wish to be treated. She has been able to communicate her needs to her carers from the outset of her illness.
2. A 62-year-old gentleman has been told that he will require an operation for prostate cancer. He refuses as he has a phobia of needles.
3. J has severe back pain but is anxious about the possibility of surgical intervention that might leave him paralysed. He is told by the surgeon that if that happens, he would be the first one as all his operations have been successful. Following the operation, he is paralysed from the waist down.

In considering the above-mentioned scenarios, you would have needed to consider whether

- in scenario 1, the 52-year old has capacity to refuse life saving treatment;
- in scenario 2, the phobia of needles causes temporary incapacity;
- in scenario 3, whether consent given is valid.

The issue of capacity is an important aspect of consent. The law provides that where the patient appears not to have the relevant capacity, any interventions should be carried out in the best interests of the patient. The Mental Capacity Act (2005) provides a regime that enables healthcare professionals to determine whether an individual has the relevant capacity to make healthcare decisions. This legislative measure applies to all aged 16 or over, as they are presumed to have the ability to make decisions about their own healthcare needs. The Mental Capacity Act (2005) has five guiding principles that recommends how healthcare professionals should deal with capacity/incapacity:

- A person must be assumed to have capacity unless it is established that he lacks capacity.
- A person is not to be treated as unable to make a decision unless all practicable steps to help him to do so have been taken without success.
- A person is not to be treated as unable to make a decision merely because he makes an unwise decision.
- An act done or decision made, under this Act for or on behalf of a person who lacks capacity must be done, or made, in his best interests.
- Before the act is done or the decision is made, consideration must be given as to whether the purpose for which it is needed can be as effectively achieved in a way that is less restrictive of the person's rights and freedom of action.

Any doubts as to the incapacity of the individual to make the relevant decision needs to be assessed. The Mental Capacity Act (2005) provides a two-stage functional test based on the decision that needs to be made at the time. The following questions must be asked:

- Is there a permanent or temporary impairment or disturbance to the functioning of the mind or brain?
- And if so, how does the impairment affect the ability of the person to make the decision?

The statutory test for capacity is found in Section 3 MCA (2005), which provides that

'(1) a person is unable to make a decision for himself if he is unable

  a. to understand the information relevant to the decision,
  b. to retain that information,
  c. tuse or weigh that information as part of the process of making the decision, or
  d. to communicate his decision (whether by talking, using sign language or any other means)'.

Any question of capacity is to be determined on a balance of probabilities.

In relation to patients receiving palliative care, seeking consent prior to treatment is important primarily because capacity may fluctuate. Patients may well evaluate the necessity of undergoing a treatment regime that is palliative rather than curative.

Activity 4.3

Jane is undergoing both radiotherapy and chemotherapy treatment. It is proposed to offer her further chemotherapy in a last ditch attempt to halt the spread of cancer. At first Jane was happy to agree to any treatment proposed but recently she has been feeling down. She is tearful and has begun to question the purpose of all the treatment. She is finding it difficult to manage the side effects from the radiotherapy and chemotherapy. She is tired of taking all these pills as she says. She is now refusing to undergo this last round of radiotherapy and chemotherapy. Discuss whether Jane has the relevant capacity to refuse the proposed treatment

---

In considering the above activity, you would need to assess her capacity as she may be suffering from depression that may prevent her from making the right decision; that is, the depression will trigger the assessment which will lead to the two-stage functional test.

In some cases, others may be designated to make a decision on behalf of another adult. The Mental Capacity Act (2005) has two formal powers that allow a third party to make decisions on behalf of another person. These powers permit the designated person to consent or refuse medical treatment. The powers are as follows:

- Health and welfare LPA
  This allows another person to consent on behalf of a person who lacks capacity. The LPA has to have been granted by the person when they had capacity and comes into force only when they lose capacity. The LPA needs to be registered with the office of Public Guardian.
- Court of protection deputy
  Where continuing decisions needs to be made for the treatment of an incapable patient and there is no LPA, the Court of protection may appoint a deputy to make health and welfare decisions on the person's behalf that can include the right to consent or refuse treatment.

In addition, the Mental Capacity Act (2005) also allows for individuals to make an advance decision to refuse treatment. Sections 24–26 of the MCA give statutory recognition to advance decisions refusing treatment and specify the conditions that must be fulfilled before such a decision or directive is considered to be valid and applicable. An advance decision is a decision to refuse specified treatment in the future, which is effective when the person loses the capacity to consent or refuse treatment.

An advance directive is valid if

- it is made by a person aged 18 or over;
- it is made at the time the patient has capacity;
- it specifies the treatment that they do not wish to receive.

An advance directive may be withdrawn at any time and need not be in writing (Box 4.3).

An advance decision is not applicable if

- the patient is capable of giving or refusing consent to the treatment proposed at the time;
- the treatment proposed is not covered by the advance decision;

Box 4.3 Case study: HE v A Hospital NHS Trust 2003 2 FLR 408

A woman who suffered from a congenital heart problem had made an advance directive refusing blood products at a time when she was a practicing Jehovah's witness. She had subsequently become engaged to a Muslim and was professing that she would abide by the principles of that faith when she was taken seriously ill and rushed to hospital. Her father applied to the court for an order that the hospital give her a blood transfusion to save her life, as the advance decisions no longer reflected her intentions. The Court held that the advance directive was no longer valid as the assumption on which the advance directive was based has been destroyed by the abandonment of her faith as a Jehovah's witness. The Advance directive need not be expressly revoked.

- the circumstances to which the decisions are based on are absent;
- there are reasonable grounds to believe that the patient may not have taken into consideration circumstances or factors if known at the time that they would not have led to the advance directive.

Sections 25 (5) & (6) of the MCA provide additional safeguards in relation to life-sustaining treatment. They are as follows:

- the patient must state that the refusal for a specific treatment is to be complied with even if life is at risk;
- the statement must be in writing and signed by the patient or another person in the patient's presence and by the patient's direction;
- be witnessed.

Improvements in life expectancy mean living longer. The Centre for Population Change (2010) suggests that 2.1% of UK residents are currently aged 85 and over, which may raise the issue of who will make decisions on behalf of a person who lacks capacity and has no one to advocate on their behalf. The MCA (2005) has incorporated a 'duty to instruct' before providing 'serious medical treatment' to a patient who lacks capacity and there is no one with whom the provider of treatment can discuss the nature of the treatment with. The duty to instruct an independent mental capacity advocate (IMCA) only applies where serious medical treatment is being considered. This includes treatment that involves providing, withdrawing or withholding treatment in circumstances where there is a fine balance to be drawn between the benefits and risks associated with the treatment, or alternatively there is a choice of treatments or the treatment proposed involves serious consequences for the patient. The IMCA will be entitled to have access to any health record, social services record or care home record, which may be relevant to the investigation. The IMCA following consultation will then make a recommendation to the provider as to what should be done (Box 4.4).

Box 4.4 Case study: IMCA referral taken from The involvement of IMCAs in serious medical treatment available at www.actionforadvocacy.org.uk p20

Sarah is a 35-year-old woman with learning difficulties. She communicates largely through gestures and pictures and those who know her have developed a good understanding of her needs based on her behaviour and communication methods. Sarah has been prescribed Clonazepam for some years for epilepsy and generally remains well, although occasionally refuses to take the medication when she experiences changes in her home life. Recently her seizures have increased; this is demonstrated on a recording chart the residential care home staff keeps in Sarah's notes. Sarah's care team arranges a visit to the GP to discuss this, who suggests a blood test to check the levels of Clonazepam to determine the efficacy of the medication. Sarah is deemed not to have the capacity to consent to the blood test, as she is unable to weigh or understand its purpose. Although this would normally be viewed as a routine procedure, which the GP can carry out in Sarah's best interests, Sarah becomes very distressed when he tries to examine her, becoming tearful and hitting out at the GP. The GP, therefore, determines that a best interests meeting needs to take place to discuss the potential options, including sedation, as well as the risks, benefits and burdens of each option.

An IMCA needs to be instructed, as Sarah has no family or friends to represent her. The IMCA quickly commences their work and meets with Sarah, examines relevant records including both health and social care, consults with those that provide care in Sarah's home as well as asks relevant questions about the risks, benefits and burdens within each option presented. The IMCA submits a report that is balanced in terms of both highlighting the risks and benefits of each option as well as identifying the least restrictive option and advocating Sarah's wishes.

Best interests

Any decision made on behalf of the patient who lacks capacity needs to be made in his or her best interests. The concept of 'best interests' are wider than just medical best interests. Section 4 of the MCA provides a detailed framework for assessment of best interests. These are as follows:

- All relevant circumstances must be taken into account and these may include, for example, religious beliefs and known wishes.
- Reasonable steps to be taken to ensure that the person to whom the decision applies is encouraged and enabled to participate. This may involve providing treatment or therapies to encourage communication.
- Previously held beliefs and feelings. The family and close friends may be a source of those views and opinions.
- Not to be motivated to bring about the death of the person.
- Consider alternative options for treatment.

Withholding and withdrawing treatment

There is a prima facie duty to take reasonable steps to keep the patient alive but only if it is clinically indicated. The withdrawal or withholding of treatment is an issue that confronts healthcare professionals in a palliative setting. As palliative care is aimed at the prevention of or the minimization of distressing symptoms, at some point a decision will need to be made as to whether treatment should be withheld or withdrawn. The difficulty lies in the prediction of death and the intention to cause death. The law is clear that it is unlawful to intentionally cause the death of a person, but recognizes the situation where treatment is good and that there is a sufficient balance of good over potential harmful effects, for example, in the use of pain killing drugs that may shorten life. The principle of double effect applies where the unintended effect of treatment shortens the life of the patient. Furthermore, there are situations where the withdrawal of treatment may bring about the death of the patient such as the withdrawal of artificial nutrition and hydration or the withdrawal of ventilation. In such cases, a declaration by the court will need to be sought prior to the withdrawal unless an advance directive is in place (Box 4.5 and Box 4.6).

Box 4.5 Case study: the doctrine of double effect: Mr. Justice Devlin in R v Bodkin Adams, 1957

Mr. Justice Devlin said: 'if the purpose of medicine, the restoration of health, can no longer be achieved there is still much for a doctor to do, and **he is entitled to do all that is proper and necessary to relieve pain and suffering, even if the measures he takes may incidentally shorten life ...** "cause" means nothing philosophical or technical or scientific. It means what you twelve men and women sitting as a jury in the jury box would regard in a common-sense way as the cause ... But, it remains the law, that no doctor, nor any man, no more in the case of the dying man than of the healthy, has the right deliberately to cut the thread of life'.

Box 4.6 Case study: withdrawing treatment in a patient in a permanent vegetative state: the case of bland (Airedale NHS trust v Bland, 1993) and guidance to health care staff

In 1989, Anthony Bland was seriously hurt following the Hillsborough football disaster. Attempts to resuscitate Bland led him to be in a persistent vegetative state. He was in this state for 3 years before his parents asked whether treatment could be withdrawn to allow him to die. The trust applied to the court for a ruling as to whether it would be lawful to discontinue Bland's artificial nutrition and hydration. The House of Lords's decision was important in three respects.

- It clarified the legal position with regard to a doctor withholding or withdrawing treatment from a patient who is in a permanent vegetative state.
- It established that nutrition and hydration is part of medical treatment.
- It made a significant contribution to the legal position with regard to advance directives (now enshrined in the MCA 2005).

Do not resuscitate orders (DNR)

Hospitals, general practices, residential care homes and ambulance services are required to have policies regarding cardio pulmonary resuscitation (CPR) that respect patients' rights. CPR could be applied to anyone prior to death, but clearly, it is important to identify those patients in whom death is imminent and for whom CPR would be inappropriate. However, decisions not to resuscitate are an emotive issue, which will require careful and sensitive handling with relatives and next-of-kins. The review of the LCP highlighted some of the issues in relation to DNRs where, for example, relatives were not consulted. It is important, therefore, that the patient is consulted if possible as well as the family.

Activity 4.4

R is a 34-year-old man with cerebral palsy whose condition was deteriorating both neurologically and physically. He has had numerous chest infections, severe constipation and bleeding from an ulcerated oesophagus. Dr. S has signed a 'DNR'. You are concerned about the legality of the 'DNR'. What steps would you take should you wish to challenge the appropriateness of the 'DNR'?

In considering the above activity you would need to be aware of the following:

- the policies in relation to the imposition of a 'DNR';
- the condition of R;
- known wishes of R;
- has the family been consulted?
- should the provider seek a declaration from the Court?

Euthanasia and assisted suicide

Euthanasia is defined as the painless killing of a patient suffering from an incurable and painful disease or is in an irreversible coma. The advent of technological advances has increased our ability to prolong life where in the past it would not have been possible. This ability to prolong life has meant that some have questioned whether it is a good thing to prolong life, particularly, if the quality of life is likely to be poor. The legal position relevant to end of life decisions in a clinical context is set out in the following:

- Active euthanasia is unlawful whether voluntary or not. Any steps taken to actively shorten the life of a patient amounts to murder. For example, injecting the patient with potassium chloride which has no pain relieving agents will be deemed unlawful.
- Passive euthanasia on the other hand is not necessarily unlawful if the reasons for withdrawing treatment is made on sound clinical reasoning and is in the best interests of the patient. It is noted here that any decision to withhold or withdraw treatment could be challenged in court. The court would need to decide whether the withholding or withdrawing of treatment was negligent. In doing so, the court would apply the Bolam test, that is, whether the doctor fell below *the standard of the ordinary skilled man exercising and professing to have that special skill. A man need not possess the highest expert skill at the risk of being found negligent. It is well established law that it is sufficient if he exercises the ordinary skill of an ordinary man exercising that particular art* (Bolam v Friern Hospital management committee, 1957).
- Assisted suicide is unlawful in the United Kingdom (s2 Suicide Act 1961); that said, there is ongoing debate about the legalisation of assisted suicide. Lord Joffe, in 2006, proposed a Bill that would permit a doctor to prescribe a lethal dose of medication that the patient could take themselves but the House of Lords blocked the bill. Since then the media has reported a number of UK citizens who have travelled to Switzerland to bring their lives to an end. There have been two challenges to the right to die in the UK courts [see case studies in Box 4.7, Box 4.8, Box 4.9 and Box 4.10, in following text]. The issue of assisted suicide is particularly an emotive one, which sees the public divided whether legalisation of assisted should be permitted or not. Doctors, back in 2006, were surveyed by the UK Royal College of physicians and by the BMA, who found a high proportion opposing the legalisation of assisted suicide. Recently, The Independent MSP Margo Macdonald put forward a bill in the Scottish parliament to legalise assisted suicide. This was rejected by the Scottish parliament by 85 votes to 16 with two abstentions. In 2010, following a number of legal challenges by Debbie Purdy, the Department of Public prosecutions (DPP), stated that there had been no change in the law but issued guidelines in relation to the manner in which it exercises its discretion not to prosecute. The DPP will publish the facts and circumstances he takes into consideration when deciding whether to prosecute or not:

Box 4.7 16 public interest factors in favour of prosecution

- The victim was under 18 years of age.
- The victim did not have the capacity (as defined by the Mental Capacity Act 2005) to reach an informed decision to commit suicide.
- The victim had not reached a voluntary, clear, settled and informed decision to commit suicide.
- The victim had not clearly and unequivocally communicated his or her decision to commit suicide to the suspect.
- The victim did not seek the encouragement or assistance of the suspect personally or on his or her own initiative.

- The suspect was not wholly motivated by compassion; for example, the suspect was motivated by the prospect that he or she or a person closely connected to him or her stood to gain in some way from the death of the victim.
- The suspect pressured the victim to commit suicide.
- The suspect did not take reasonable steps to ensure that any other person had not pressured the victim to commit suicide.
- The suspect had a history of violence or abuse against the victim.
- The victim was physically able to undertake the act that constituted the assistance to him or herself.
- The suspect was unknown to the victim and encouraged or assisted the victim to commit or attempt to commit suicide by providing specific information via, for example, a website or publication.
- The suspect gave encouragement or assistance to more than one victim who was not known to each other.
- The suspect was paid by the victim or those close to the victim for his or her encouragement or assistance.
- The suspect was acting in his or her capacity as a medical doctor, nurse, other healthcare professional, a professional carer (whether for payment or not), or as a person in authority, such as a prison officer, and the victim was in his or her care.
- The suspect was aware that the victim intended to commit suicide in a public place where it was reasonable to think that members of the public may be present.
- The suspect was acting in his or her capacity as a person involved in the management or as an employee (whether for payment or not) of an organisation or group, a purpose of which is to provide a physical environment (whether for payment or not) in which to allow another to commit suicide.

Box 4.8 6 public interest factors against prosecution

- The victim had reached a voluntary, clear, settled and informed decision to commit suicide.
- The suspect was wholly motivated by compassion.
- The actions of the suspect, although sufficient to come within the definition of the crime, were of only minor encouragement or assistance.
- The suspect had sought to dissuade the victim from taking the course of action which resulted in his or her suicide.
- The actions of the suspect may be characterised as reluctant encouragement or assistance in the face of a determined wish on the part of the victim to commit suicide.
- The suspect reported the victim's suicide to the police and fully assisted them in their enquiries into the circumstances of the suicide or the attempt and his or her part in providing encouragement or assistance.

Box 4.9 Case study : landmark victory for Debbie Purdy available at www.theguardian.com 30 July 2009

Debbie Purdy won a landmark victory in securing a review of the law on assisted suicide. Purdy, 45, wants her husband, Omar Puente, to accompany her to the Dignitas clinic in Switzerland to end her life once her suffering has become unbearable. However, she was worried he could be prosecuted on returning to the United Kingdom. Puente would be liable to prosecution and a prison term of up to 14 years if found guilty of assisting, aiding or abetting a suicide. Lord Justice Latham, sitting with Mr Justice Nelson at the high court in London, ruled that "without wishing to give Ms Purdy any optimism that her arguments will ultimately succeed", she did have an arguable case which should go to a full hearing. It is currently illegal in the United Kingdom to assist the suicide of another person – even if it happens abroad and assisted suicide is legal in that country. But the legal situation was unclear, because none of the relatives of the 92 Britons who have already died at Dignitas have been prosecuted on their return to the United Kingdom. Since then the DPP has clarified its guidelines on assisted suicide law (see boxes 4.7 and 4.8).

Box 4.10 Case study: R (purdy) v DPP 2002

Diane Pretty suffered from motor neurone disease and was paralysed from the neck downwards. She wanted to choose her moment of death but she was not able to bring her own life to an end as a result of her disability. She wished her husband to aid her. The Director of Public Prosecutions, however, refused to give an assurance that her husband would not be prosecuted for the offence of assisting her in her suicide under section 2 (1) of the Suicide Act 1961. She challenged the refusal of the DPP. The case was heard both in the House of Lords and then the European Court of Human Rights who refused to overturn the DPP's decision to grant immunity from prosecution. Their reasons for doing so can be summarized as follows:

- No right to choose whether to live or die.
- Reasserted the principle of sanctity of life.
- The convention of human rights does not guarantee a right to assisted suicide.
- The blanket ban on assisted suicide under the suicide Act 1961 was not disproportionate.

Verification of death

Verification of death is defined as deciding whether a patient is actually dead. Nurses are now permitted to verify that the patient has died but they are not permitted legally to certify death. The Nursing Midwifery Council (2006) states that *a registered nurse may confirm or verify life extinct providing there is an explicit local protocol in place to allow such an action, which includes guidance on when other authorities, e.g. the police or the coroner, should be informed prior to the removal of the body*. Nurses are advised to comply with their local protocols on verification of death but as a rule, nurses should only verify death in circumstances where death is expected. Expected death is defined as *death where a patients demise is anticipated in the near future and the doctor will be able to issue a medical certificate as to the cause of death (i.e. the doctor has seen the patient within the last 14 days before the death)* (Home Office 1971). In order for nurses to carry out this task, they must receive appropriate training so that they be confident in interpreting and applying the local policy.

Conclusion

An overview of the main legal issues associated with palliative care has been discussed. The activities and case studies set out in the chapter are designed to enable the reader to provide care for patients in a palliative setting that is in line with the legal requirements. It is not intended to give you a solution to the issues raised in the palliative context, rather it is intended to help you practise within a legal framework. It is hoped that you will have derived sufficient understanding of what the main issues are coupled with the relevant knowledge of law.

Glossary

Advance directive	A statement of a patient's wish to refuse a particular type of medical treatment or care if they become unable to make or communicate decisions for themselves.
Artificial nutrition and hydration	clinically assisted nutrition and hydration by tube or drip.
Capacity	The ability to make a decision.
Do not resuscitate order	Advanced management plan that means that a doctor is not required to resuscitate a patient if their heart stops.
Legal proxy	A person with legal authority to make certain decisions on behalf of another adult.
Verification of death	Process by which the death of a patient is established.

References

Airedale NHS trust v Bland (1993) 1 ALL 821 HL

Bolam v Friern Hospital Management Committee (1957) 1 WLR 582.

Centre for Population Change (2010). *Demographic Issues, Projections and Trends: Older People with High Support Needs in the UK.*

Department for constitutional affairs (2007). *Mental Capacity Act 2005 Section 3 (1), Section 4, Section 25 (5) & (6), Sections 24–26*. London: Stationery office.

HE v A Hospital NHS Trust (2003) 2 FLR 408
Hirsch, A. (2009) *Landmark Victory for Debbie Purdy*. Available at www.theguardian.com [accessed 17 February 2014].
Home Office (1971) *Report of the Committee on Death Certification and Coroners, Nov: Cmnd 4810*
IMCA (2010) referral taken from *The Involvement of IMCAs in Serious Medical Treatment*. Available at www.actionforadvocacy.org.uk p20 [accessed 17 February 2014].
Nursing Midwifery Council (2006) *Advice Sheet on Death Certification*. London: NMC.
Pretty v UK (2002) 35 ECHR (European court of Human Rights) application number 2346/02
RE MB (caesarian section [1997] CA) 2 FLR 426
R v Bodkin Adams (1957). *Criminal Law Review* 365
Schloendorff v Society of New York hospitals (1914) 211 NY 125
Suicide Act (1961) Section 2 (1). Available at www.legislation.gov.uk [accessed 17 February 2014].
The CPS: Assisted suicide policy (2010) Available at www.cps.gov.uk [accessed 17 February 2014].
Walton, W.-J. (2009) Verification of death by nurses in community care settings *End of life care*. 3(2): 14–19.

5

Ethical principles in palliative care

Chantal Patel

Introduction

As discussed in previous chapters, palliative care aims to enhance the quality of life for both the patient and their families. It is important to note that palliative care does not seek to bring about an early death. Some situations in palliative care give rise to complex dilemmas, raising questions about whether an action is ethically justifiable. Often, the law is unlikely to provide a solution.

Learning outcomes

By the end of this chapter you will be able to

- define the term 'ethics';
- have an understanding of the two major ethical theories;
- identify ethical issues in palliative care;
- use a principle-based approach when dealing with an ethical concern relating to palliative care.

Fundamentals of Palliative Care for Student Nurses, First Edition. Megan Rosser and Helen C. Walsh.

Companion website: www.wiley.com/go/rosser_walsh/fundamentals_of_palliative_care

Activity 5.1

Consider the following situations you could find yourself involved in:

- Mrs T refuses to eat or drink as she wishes to be allowed to die;
- Mr X requests that he be given a high dose of morphine to put him out of his misery;
- The relatives of Miss B does not want her to know that she has an incurable disease.

The meaning of ethics

Ethics is a branch of philosophy concerned with determining whether an action towards a person is right or wrong. Nurses caring for patients with palliative care needs will no doubt be confronted with situations where no clear conclusion can be reached as to what should or ought to be done.

Activity 5.2

The relatives of Miss B have requested that Miss B is not told that she has an incurable disease. Miss B takes an unexpected turn for the worse and dies before her family could be with her. She became very frightened and distressed when she realised she was dying. The nurses were not able to keep her pain-free. The family asked you whether she has died peacefully. What will you tell them? Set out your reasons for either telling the truth or withholding the truth (read Jackson 1991 for further guidance on telling the truth).

Our moral compass is not only influenced by the law but by culture, religion, beliefs, values, personal conscience, personal convictions and experience. When confronted with moral issues in the clinical context, it is imperative that the issues are explored to ascertain what should be done.

In the above scenario, you may choose to withhold the truth as you may believe that it is best if the family remains ignorant of her distress and fear or alternatively you might tell the truth. Here are some thoughts on the matter that you may have considered.

Withhold the truth	Tell the truth
• It would be pointless to distress the family further by informing them of her distress and fear prior to death • The family may well find it hard to grieve her death as they may feel remorse and guilt	• The truth will be painful but lying now may cause difficulties in the future as the family is likely to be confronted with similar situations in the future

Activity 5.3

List your reasons for either telling or withholding the truth when dealing with patients, generally.

In doing so consider the following:

- Is there a duty of honesty on healthcare professionals?
- Is the duty situational?
- Is intentional deception acceptable, and if so, when is it morally defensible?
- What is the difference between an outright lie and being economical with the truth?
- Can you think of situations where it would be in the patient's best interests to be deceived?

There are a number of issues that may arise in the context of palliative care; these centre around:

- the non-curative nature of the disease;
- the relief of pain;
- treatment to alleviate symptoms;
- withholding or withdrawing of artificial hydration and nutrition;
- the agreement to undergo treatment;
- disclosure of disease to relatives.

Furthermore, in palliative care, the nurse needs to consider what their responsibilities are when caring for patients. These could be grouped as follows (Box 5.1):

Edwards (2009) describes ethics as the application of principles to a moral problem to ascertain whether an action is right or wrong. Beauchamp and Childress (1989) developed an approach to resolve moral dilemmas in healthcare based on four principles. They are as follows:

- respect for autonomy;
- beneficence;
- non-maleficence;
- justice.

Box 5.1 Nurses' responsibilities

- to provide an appropriate level of care;
- to be honest with the patient;
- to maintain confidentiality;
- to maintain appropriate relations with relatives;
- to maintain trust by managing potential conflict of interest.

Beauchamp and Childress (2001) believe that these principles cover most of the moral issues encountered in healthcare.

a. Autonomy
   Autonomy can be defined as 'self-rule', that is, the ability for an adult of sound mind to make decisions concerning their own lives. Respect for autonomy is the 'moral obligation to respect the autonomy of others in so far as such respect is compatible with equal respect for the autonomy of all potentially affected' (Gillon, 1994). In today's healthcare arena, an emphasis is placed on the importance of respecting the right of an individual to make decisions even if the decisions are not supported by nurses or doctors. In order to promote the autonomy of an individual, it is important that the relevant information is given to assist the decision making process. It would be unethical for any treatment to be given without the consent of the individual. However, in a palliative environment it can be difficult to ascertain whether the choices made are as a result of an appropriate understanding of the circumstances the individual finds himself or herself in. Care needs to be taken to ensure that any decision made is as a result of careful weighing up of all the relevant information.

Activity 5.4

James is a 34-year-old man who has been diagnosed with testicular cancer. Surgery is planned and it is expected to be successful. James has a learning disability and lives in a residential setting. James has a limited understanding of his condition. He does, however, understand that he will need to undergo an operation. He has said that he does not wish to have the operation even if that means he may die.

Should James wish be respected? And, if so, what would have influenced you in respecting his wishes?

In determining whether James' wishes should be respected, you may have considered the following:

- His capacity in relation to his condition, that is, James understands the consequences of not having the operation including potential distress of managing an untreated condition.
- Eliciting the reasons as to why James does not wish to undergo a surgical operation.
- Are there any alternatives to surgical interventions?

b. Beneficence and non-maleficence
   Beneficence and non-maleficence are normally considered together as they are often seen as two sides of the same coin. Beneficence is the duty to do good whilst non-maleficence is the duty not to harm. When providing medical treatment, there is always a potential risk of harming the patient. It is, therefore, important to assess whether any treatment provided will bring some benefit to the patient. In a non-curative arena, it is often difficult to measure what benefits treatment may bring, in particular, if the treatment is likely to be palliative.

In such cases, it is said that treatment provided should be in the best interests of the patient, that is, any treatment that is good for the patient or beneficial to the patient.

Activity 5.5

Mary, a 79-year-old lady, with end-stage heart failure has a chest infection. Mary is very frail and will imminently die. Her chest infection could be treated with antibiotics, which is likely to provide some relief. Would the administration of antibiotics be in her best interests all things considered?

---

c. Justice
The duty of justice is defined as an obligation to act on the basis of fair adjudication between competing claims. This duty is subdivided into three categories:

- Distributive justice
This involves allocation of resources on a fair basis. Medical advances have increased demands for more expensive treatment including expensive drugs on the NHS. This has led to prioritisation of care and treatment on the NHS. In 2005, the media highlighted the concerns around denial of life saving drugs as well as restrictions on access to treatment. The NHS has to ensure that it can provide a service to all within an allocated budget. Therefore, it is imperative to have a strong rationale for supporting treatment in a palliative environment. It is not that individuals are being denied treatment because their condition is non-curative, rather a view has to be taken as to whether such treatment can be sanctioned on grounds of beneficence and whether the treatment is affordable. Klein *et al.* (1996) suggested that distribution of resources is based on the exercise of reason, which is carried out fairly and even-handedly. Nevertheless in a practical context, healthcare professionals have to decide whether treatment is advocated or not. For example, the doctor may have to decide whether the use of antibiotics on a patient with chronic obstructive pulmonary disease is justified and can be withheld, in particular, if the individual refuses to pay heed to medical advice and continues to engage in activity that is detrimental to the condition. A further issue is that equality is at the heart of justice. Thus, to achieve a fair outcome it is important to treat equals equally and unequals unequally. However, debate regarding the morally relevant criteria when deciding to treat people as equals or unequals continues to this date. We are no closer to finding agreement than we were when Aristotle first discussed the issue of equality. The best we can do is to manage each patient based on their clinical needs with the support of their next of kin/carer. Here, the healthcare professional needs to be careful that they do not impose their own personal or professional views about justice on others. Any decision to withhold or withdraw treatment must be thought through and in doing so the healthcare professional needs to be aware of the following:

  - conflicts may exist between several common moral concerns;
  - provision of sufficient healthcare to meet the needs of all who need it;

Box 5.2 Case Study – Postcode lottery for cancer wonder drug (mail Online April 10, 2006)

Breast cancer patients from England must pay £47000 to get the wonder drug Herceptin at the same hospital where Welsh women get it for free. All Welsh Local health Boards have agreed to pay for the drug for women living in Wales who need it even if they are treated in England, but the primary care trust in Shropshire has refused to pay for Herceptin for early stage breast cancer sufferers until the drug is licensed. As the drug has been licensed, it is now available subject to guidelines from the National Institute of Clinical Excellence. Whilst this media storm concentrated on the availability of a drug for breast cancer sufferers, it remains today that availability of some treatments are still subject to postcode lottery. For example, BBC News Online on the March 8, 2013 commented that there were stark variations in the accessibility of surgery on the NHS owing to rationing. (BBC NEWS online March 8, 2013)

- distribution of health care resources in proportion to the extent of people's needs for healthcare;
- healthcare professionals to prioritise the needs of their patients;
- provision of equal access to health care;
- allowance of choice as much as possible;
- maximisation of benefit produced by the available resources;
- respecting the autonomy of those who provide the resources (Box 5.2).

- Rights-based justice concerns the rights of individual with equal right to be treated equally, whilst those who do not have those rights should be treated unequally. For example, those who do not need medication should not get medication.
- Legal justice requires that nurses obey morally acceptable laws. For example, there are rules in relation to maintaining confidentiality that you may not agree with but any breach will be subject to sanctions.

Activity 5.6

Justice

Marina, an 18-year-old, has been diagnosed with a rare form of cancer for which there is a new drug on the market but the efficacity of the drug is only 50%. Esther, a 79-year-old, has breast cancer and the treatment available offers a chance of 80% to 90% success. The resources available will only permit the treatment of one person. Who will you support: Marina or Esther? Give your reasons for the decision you make.

Activity 5.7

Applying the four principles

Max is 19-years old. He has recently been diagnosed with non-Hodgkin's Lymphoma. He is refusing to undergo conventional treatment which has shown to be very effective. Max prefers to opt for homeopathic treatment, which includes regular coffee enemas. His mum is very worried and would like Max to be given the treatment to maximise his chances of survival. His mum states that Max is a little immature and tends to be swayed by literature he reads on natural health. She asserts that Max does not understand the consequences of not accepting conventional treatment.

Consider whether Max should be forced to undergo conservative treatment despite his refusal?

In considering the above scenario, you should consider the following:

- Respect for Max's autonomy
  To maximise Max's ability to make the right decision, we should give Max all the relevant information to promote and respect his autonomy. Max's views need to be considered carefully to assess whether Max has the relevant ability to make the decision he is about to embark upon. Has Max considered the consequences of his refusal for treatment? Does he have an understanding of the level of distress and potential suffering? Max's decision can only be respected if the decision is made by a competent adult. We can only be sure of this if he fully understands the consequences that may flow from his decision.

- Beneficence
  The role of nurses is to act in the best interests of their patients. This may conflict with the principle of autonomy. Max has indicated his refusal, which from a professional standpoint may not be in his best interest. The treatment proposed is known to be effective and it is appropriate for healthcare professionals to take into consideration both the long-term and short-term impact of overriding Max's view. A short-term impact may lead to a breakdown in the trust placed in healthcare professionals as well as a potential refusal to seek medical treatment. It may also lead to a breakdown in his relationship with his mum at a time that he most needs it. The long-term impact suggests that Max's condition is likely to be beneficial as without treatment, Max's chances of survival are reduced. The benefits of acting in Max's best interests against his wishes will need to be weighed against the failure to respect Max's refusal to undergo the relevant treatment as indicated. It is necessary to point out here that from a legal standpoint, Max, if assessed as a competent adult, cannot be forced to undergo any treatment.

- Non-maleficence
  There is a duty on healthcare professionals not to inflict harm to their patients. Max is likely to be harmed if forced to undergo treatment against his wishes but without the treatment,

Max is unlikely to survive. Which action is likely to result in the greatest harm? In considering this aspect, a number of assumptions will need to be made, for example, how successful will the treatment be and how will Max be willing to comply with treatment.

- Justice
  Whilst an emphasis is placed on the right of an individual to make decisions that matter to them and their life plans, it is relevant to consider the potential impact on the health service. One needs to consider whether there will be complications arising out of his refusal to undergo conventional treatment and opting for homeopathic treatment instead. Will any subsequent treatment be more costly?

The principle-based approach as advocated by Beauchamp and Childress concerns a framework that allows you to justify why you would advocate a particular approach. Gillon (1994) stated that the best moral strategy he has found when dealing with ethical dilemmas was to distinguish between whether he was being asked to make a decision or whether he was expected to make a decision on behalf of the organisation or profession. For example, you may have a personal view on withdrawal of treatment, but what is the organisational/professional/societal view on withdrawal of treatment. In dealing with ethical dilemmas as a nurse you should aim to

- exclude any decisions or views that have no moral justification, for example, withholding antibiotics to smokers who refuse to give up smoking;
- to use all resources available cost effectively;
- to respect patient's rights;
- to obey morally acceptable laws.

Notwithstanding our commitment to provide care that is morally justifiable, we need to recognise that there is scope to disagree on the appropriate application of the principle-based approach to moral dilemmas. For example, to whom do we owe these moral obligations? For nurses, our actions are guided by the special relationship we have with our patients but there are two issues of practical importance which needs to be considered:

- the obligation of respect for autonomy and to whom it applies;
- the scope of a 'right to life' as well as a 'right to die'.

Ethical theories

In addition to the principle-based approach, there are two major ethical theories that guide healthcare practice.

Deontology

A duty-based theory which holds there is a duty to act in accordance with a set of universal moral rules regardless of the consequences. For example, deontologists hold views such as

- it is wrong to kill innocent people;
- it is wrong to tell lies;
- it is right to keep promises.

The Nursing and Midwifery Council's code of conduct (2008) for its registrants imposes various duties, inter alia:

- make the care of people your first concern, treating them as individuals and respecting their dignity;
- work with others to protect and promote the health and well-being of those in your care, their families and carers, and the wider community;
- provide a high standard of practice and care at all times;
- be open and honest, act with integrity and uphold the reputation of your profession.

The language used in the code is based on this deontological concept. It assumes that every professional should act in a manner that focuses on their duty to do the right thing rather than on the consequences. The duties are based on moral rules that are universalisable. For example, is it morally permissible to break a promise? To test this, one can ask whether we should have a universal rule that says it is fine to break promises. It would be nonsensical to have a rule that permits breach of promises; therefore, it would be wrong to break promises. Any rule that cannot be universalised would not be a valid moral rule.

Activity 5.8

Consider the request by a family member that you should withhold the truth in relation to the patient's condition, for example, not divulging that the patient has an incurable illness. Map out all the potential issues in either divulging or withholding the nature of the illness to the patient. Examine how a duty-based approach will help you determine whether you will withhold the truth of the patient's condition as directed by the patient's family.

As with any major ethical theories, the duty-based approach is not without its critics, the following outlines the major criticisms associated with this theoretical approach:

- no guidance as to how to deal with potential conflict between or among the various duties;
- too rigid or absolutist, it does not allow exceptions;
- the universalisation of the rules does not necessarily point to the moral nature of the rules;
- allows acts that make the world a less good place because it is not interested in results.

Utilitarianism

A consequence-based theory holds that actions are right or wrong according to the consequences. The right act is one that produces the best overall result from an objective standpoint. This approach gives weight to the interests of all affected. The most well-known consequence-based theory, utilitarianism, focuses on one basic principle of ethics, that is , the principle of utility. This approach suggests that all actions should be assessed in terms of their overall maximal value.

Activity 5.9

Live donation of kidney

Gemma, aged 13, is in need of a kidney. Her parents and siblings are being assessed as potential donors. The blood results show that Gemma's father (Peter) is best placed to donate his organ. Peter is the sole breadwinner for the family as Gemma's mum is unable to work because of mental health problems. Gemma's father, however, is hesitant as to whether he should donate.

Consider the reasons for and against donation of organ from Peter's perspective using a utilitarian approach.

In considering the above activity, here is a non-exhaustive list of reasons for and against you might have come up with before deciding what should be done.

For	Against
• Best interests of Gemma as donation will shorten her suffering and distress if she were to wait for an organ on the waiting list • Positive impact on the family of his altruistic donation of organ to his daughter • Peter is histocompatible and surgery can take place without delay	• Peter is fearful of surgery • The possibility that transplantation may not be successful • Fear of losing his job • Fear of financial ruin • The prospect of Gemma receiving a cadaver organ

The adoption of a utilitarian approach may well lead you to the conclusion that Peter should donate his organ given the overall value to the family as well as to Gemma. While this may seem appropriate, primarily because it is simple and it appeals to common sense, some of the criticisms surrounding this approach centre on the appropriateness of the preferences that guide us as to whether an act is morally justifiable or not. Utilitarians adopt either an approach that deals with particular acts, in particular, circumstances or alternatively adopt rules that justifies actions. These are explained below (Box 5.3).

Box 5.3

Rule utilitarianism	Act utilitarianism
Focuses on moral rules, that is, the rule utilitarian considers the consequences of generally observing a rule	Focuses on the particular act. The act utilitarian is confronted by the question, 'What should I do now?'

Some criticisms of utilitarianism:

- future consequences are difficult to predict;
- difficulty in measuring the 'goodness' of consequences;
- bias in favour of particular groups;
- tendency to ignore things that we may regard as ethically relevant, for example, the character of the person doing the act is irrelevant;
- it disregards the 'fairness' of the result so long as it produces the maximum total happiness;
- it could lead to inconsistency with human rights.

Below are a number of scenarios; consider how the different utilitarian approach will determine what is the right action to take.

Activity 5.10

Scenario	Act utilitarian	Rule utilitarian
A says he will fund 1000 hip/knee replacements for the next 10 years if he is given the next available organ. This will mean that the person on top of the list is likely to die but 1000 patients will be happy with their new hips/knees.		
James is histocompatible for kidney organ donation to his son. He tells you that he does not wish to donate his organ but does not want his family to know. He asks you to tell his family that he is not histocompatible. Do you comply with his request to lie to his family?		
Jessica has been diagnosed with breast cancer. Herceptin is available but the hospital has run out of funds this year for Herceptin. If they sanction the use of Herceptin for Jessica, they will need to delay the commissioning of hip replacements by a year for at least 10 patients who have been on the waiting list for the past 6 months.		
Cynthia has ovarian cancer. She is currently receiving palliative care in a hospice. She is experiencing acute difficulty in breathing. The team decides that she will be best cared for in intensive care. Her family disagrees as they believe that she has suffered enough and it is not in her interest to keep her alive.		

When providing palliative care, the nurse may well be confronted with a variety of terms and concepts, it is important to have an understanding of these terms in order to assist the decision-making process.

- The primary goal of medicine
  Identifying the primary goal of medicine allows us as healthcare professionals to determine whether the treatment is beneficial or not. There is an assumption in healthcare that the primary goal of medicine is to restore or maintain the patient's health as far as is practicable. If this is the case, then it allows us to determine the point at which treatment can be withdrawn as any treatment is unlikely to restore or maintain the patient's health. It is noted, however, that good quality care should continue.

- Life-prolonging treatment
  This term refers to any treatment likely to postpone the patient's death. This includes, for example, cardiopulmonary resuscitation and any other specialised treatments such as chemotherapy or antibiotics. The controversy surrounding the Liverpool care pathway established in the 1990s demonstrates the difficulty in dealing with withdrawal of life-prolonging treatment.

- Capacity and incapacity
  To proceed with any treatment, consent for any interventions need to be sought from the patient undergoing the treatment. The emphasis on the right of the individual to determine for themselves what happens to their bodies is supported in law, but this right is predicated on the individual having the capacity to make the relevant decision. Assessing capacity can be difficult, in particular, as the individual may place a high importance on issues that are not medically relevant, for example, making decisions in line with their cultural or religious views. In contrast, a duty is placed on the healthcare professional to provide any necessary treatment to the best interests of the individual who does not have the relevant capacity to make the decision.

- Duty of care
  There is a moral as well as a legal obligation to take reasonable steps to keep the patient alive and to provide treatment that is clinically indicated.

- Quality of life
  It is accepted that the term 'quality of life' can be difficult to define but whichever way this is used, the term cannot be avoided when discussions centre on life-prolonging treatment. Human life has intrinsic worth and, therefore, it would be wrong to determine whether one person lives or is allowed to die on the basis of quality of life. What may be deemed to be poor quality of life to us as healthcare professionals may not be so for others. This is an issue that confronts healthcare staff whenever decisions have to be made as to whether to continue to provide treatment or withdraw treatment which effectively will shorten the life of that person. What is necessary is that the healthcare team focuses on the value of the treatment for the patient.

- Best interests
  It is a term that is used to present a reassuring standard by which decisions are made in the context of a patient who does not have the relevant capacity. This concept goes beyond medical interests; other interests such as personal wishes/values, cultural and religious views are as important.

- Futility
  Any treatment deemed unable to produce the desired benefit, that is, the treatment is unable to provide an acceptable quality of life. The difficulty with this term is that some treatment may provide short-term relief, but have no long-term benefits and as such the use of this term should be avoided given the broad definition of benefit.

- Artificial hydration and nutrition
  This refers to the provision of nutrition and hydration via nasogastric tube, percutaneous endoscopic gastrostomy (PEG feeding) and total parenteral nutrition. There is a difference of opinion as to whether artificial hydration and nutrition should be regarded as part and parcel of basic care whilst others see it as medical treatment. The latter interpretation means that a decision to withdraw can be made.

- Foresight and intention
  It is the case that healthcare professionals may predict that withholding or withdrawing treatment may result in the death of the patient. A distinction needs to be drawn between actively seeking to end the patient's life and the withdrawal of treatment which is not in the best interests of the patient.

- Withholding and withdrawing treatment
  Withholding treatment occurs when no treatment is provided, whereas withdrawing occurs after treatment has already been initiated. There is no moral or legal difference between withholding or withdrawing treatment given that the aim of providing treatment is to benefit the patient. However, healthcare professionals need to be mindful of their duty of care and as such it is morally safer to withdraw than withhold treatment (see BMA 2008 for further guidance on withholding and withdrawing treatment).

- Conscientious objection
  Health professionals are not obligated to provide treatment that goes against their conscience or clinical judgment.

Euthanasia

No discussion in relation to end-of-life issues would be complete without something being said about euthanasia. Euthanasia means 'good death' and is referred as 'mercy killing', that is, there is an intention to bring about the death of a human being either through an act or omission for the benefit of the patient. The intention to bring about the death of a human being is tantamount to murder and therefore, unlawful. Euthanasia can be categorised as active or passive, voluntary or involuntary. The decision to prematurely shorten the life of a patient may arise either where the patient refuses further treatment or life-prolonging treatment is withdrawn. The latter is done through intentional omission (not to be confused with the withholding or withdrawing of treatment considered futile). The patient essentially dies as a result of the medical condition from which he or she suffers. For example, where cardiopulmonary resuscitation is not carried out or where antibiotics are not given because of the general condition of the patient. What is crystal clear is that we are not permitted to actively terminate the life of the patient by, for example, giving a high dose of pain relieving drugs. What we are permitted to do is to give sufficient pain relieving medication that keeps the patient pain free. Examples of the difference between active and passive euthanasia are listed below ; Cox v Winchester (1992) and Airedale NHS Trust v Bland (1993) (Box 5.4).

Box 5.4 Case study – Cox, R v (1992) Winchester Crown Court, Ognall J (for lillian Boyes). Airedale NHS Trust v Bland [1993] HL	
Lillian Boyes (active euthanasia)	**Tony Bland (passive euthanasia)**
Lillian Boyes had been suffering from intractable pain because of rheumatoid arthritis, which her doctor Nigel Cox found unable to control with analgesics. She repeatedly begged him to end her life in the face of his inability to control the pain. He administered a lethal injection of potassium chloride.	Tony Bland was in a persistent vegetative state for more than 3 years. Tony could have gone on to live for 30 years or more so long as he received appropriate feeding and care. The parents sought a declaration from the courts that it would be lawful for the medical staff to withdraw feeding and other life sustaining measures so that he be allowed to die.
Dr. Cox was found guilty of attempted murder as potassium chloride was not considered to have analgesic properties. Had Dr. Cox given her an opiate, he would probably not have been tried for attempted murder.	

Euthanasia is a controversial and emotionally charged topic that polarises the public's views. Numerous attempts made to legalise the ending of a patient's life on request in parliament has failed. The main arguments for and against euthanasia are set out below.

For	Against
• Advocates of euthanasia argue that there is a moral duty to alleviate extreme pain and distress in the sufferer who wishes to die • It allows for a more dignified death in light of a poor quality of life • It allows for freedom to determine the moment of death	• It devalues human life to a mere commodity and goes against the doctrine of sanctity of life • Beauchamp and Childress (2001) highlights the potential for the 'slippery slope' effect. • The primary goal of medicine will be compromised if doctors are allowed to directly cause the death of the patient • Suspicion and mistrust may ensue if it is perceived that euthanasia is being used as a means of containing cost

Conclusion

In this chapter an overview of the ethical issues associated with palliative care has been discussed. The activities and case studies set out in the chapter are designed to enable the reader to address those practical dilemmas they may be confronted with when dealing with patients in a palliative environment. The ethical theories are not intended to give you a solution to the issues raised in the palliative context rather it is intended to help you justify your decisions supported by an appropriate ethical framework.

Glossary

Autonomy	Right to make decisions for oneself.
Beneficence	Doing good.
Best interests	Doing good for a third party who lacks capacity.
Deontology	What is right and wrong according to a set of moral duties regardless of the consequences.
Euthanasia	Painless termination of life.
Futility	Treatment that is unlikely to achieve its desired aim.
Justice	A moral obligation to be just or fair.
Non-maleficence	Doing no harm.
Utilitarianism	A consequence-based theory that holds that actions are right or wrong according to the consequences

References

Airedale NHS Trust v Bland [1993] HL

Beauchamp, T. and Childress, J. (1989) *Principles of biomedical ethics* 6th edn. Oxford university press.

Beauchamp, T. and Childress, J. (2001) *Principles of Biomedical Ethics* 5th edn. Oxford University press.

Brazier M. (2005) Commentary: an intractable dispute when parents and professionals disagree. *Medical Law Review* 13 Autumn: 412–418.

BMA (2008) *Withholding and withdrawing life prolonging treatment: guidance for decision-making* 3rd edn. Blackwell publishing.

Cox, R v (1992) Winchester Crown Court, Ognall J (for lilian Boyes).

Airedale NHS Trust v Bland [1993] HL (needs to appear in ref list as well)

Edwards, S. (2009) *Nursing ethics: A Principle Based Approach* 2nd edn. Basingstoke: Palgrave.

Gillon, R. (1994) Medical Ethics: four principles plus attention to scope. British Medical Journal. 309: 184–188.

Jackson, J. (1991) Telling the truth. *Journal of Medical Ethics* 17: 5–9.

Klein, R., Day, P. and Redmayne, S. (1996) *Managing Scarcity.* Buckingham: Open University Press.

Mail online (April 10 2006) Postcode lottery for cancer wonder drug) accessed on the 13th of March 2014 @ www.dailymail.co.uk/health/.../Postcode-lottery-cancer-wonder-drug.html

NMC (2008) *The Code: Standards of Conduct, Performance and Ethics for Nurses and Midwives* Available at www.nmc-uk.org [accessed 17 February 2014].

Wilkes, D. (2006) *Postcode Lottery for Cancer wonder Drug* Available at www.dailymail.co.uk/health/.../ Postcode-lottery-cancer-wonder-drug.ht [accessed 17 February 2014].

II

The practice of palliative care

6

Communication in palliative care

Introduction

According to Smith and Field (2011), effective communication skills are the most essential requirements of a nurse. Effective communication skills are consistently identified by patients and their families as the most important aspect of palliative care (Parker *et al*., 2007). Betcher (2010) points out that quality palliative care depends on the nurse learning about each patient and family as individuals, identifying his/her own unique needs, goals and expectations. Unless nurses use effective communication skills they are unlikely to deliver effective patient-centred quality care to this vulnerable group of patients.

Communication is a complex two-way process, which requires messages to be sent from one individual to at least one other person. These messages can relate to words, feelings or thoughts. If we do not understand the messages patients are sending, how can we accurately assess and meet their needs? More importantly, if they do not understand the messages we are sending to them, how can we expect them to co-operate in their treatment?

This chapter begins by examining the importance of communication in palliative care before exploring a simplistic, theoretical explanation of communication. The importance of self-awareness will be identified, followed by an exploration of key communication skills, the facilitators and barriers to effective communication. The chapter concludes with a brief discussion regarding the challenges of communicating with groups who have particular needs.

Fundamentals of Palliative Care for Student Nurses, First Edition. Megan Rosser and Helen C. Walsh.

Companion website: www.wiley.com/go/rosser_walsh/fundamentals_of_palliative_care

Learning outcomes

By the end of this chapter you should be able to

- identify the reasons why communication is important in palliative care;
- discuss fundamental communication theory;
- recognise the importance of self-awareness;
- identify key communication skills;
- recognise facilitators of, and barriers to, good communication; and
- consider the challenges in communicating with patients with particular needs.

Activity 6.1

Think of an occasion where you have been involved in a communication interaction with one other person. This may have occurred in a professional or social setting. What do you think made the interaction go well? Now think of a time when the communication interaction did not go so well. What made this interaction less successful? You may like to create two lists which may be similar to those in Table 6.1.

Table 6.1 Characteristics of successful and unsuccessful communication interactions.

Successful communication	Less successful communication
Appropriate non-verbal communication Good eye contact Good body language Common understanding, interest and purpose Felt, listen to and valued Common language No distractions Purpose of interaction understood and achieved Suitable environment Plenty of time No interruptions Appropriate humour Felt good afterwards Satisfactory conclusion	Other person did not seem interested Other person interrupted me Lack of eye contact Terms and words used that I did not understand Differing understanding Talked over or my point of view ignored Did not feel valued Felt rushed Felt ignored Lack of time Distracting environment Different language Defensive body language – a bit threatening No common understanding Unsatisfactory conclusion

The importance of communication in palliative care

Activity 6.2

Just spend a few minutes identifying why you think communication is important in palliative care? Jot down key words, maybe developing a mind map which you can add to as you work through the chapter. Compare your answer to the points raised in Figure 6.1.

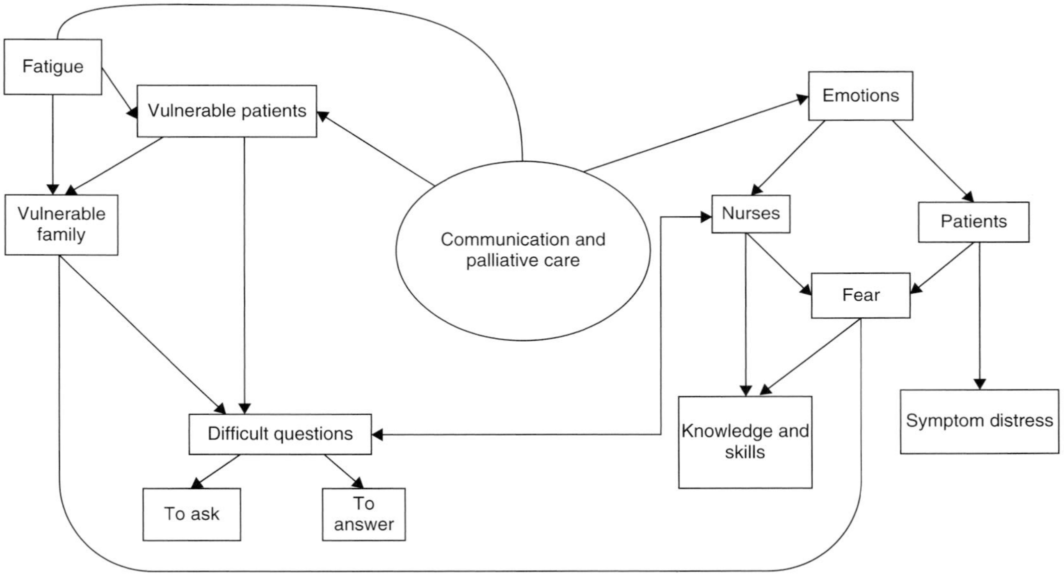

Figure 6.1 Mind map of the importance of communication in palliative care.

Of all health care professionals, nurses spend the most time with patients and it is often during times when receiving personal care that the patient may ask questions about his/her future prognosis, for example, . 'When am I going to get better?' or 'Am I dying nurse?' As the timing and nature of these questions cannot be anticipated it is difficult to plan a response in advance. If the nurse fails to respond in a way which encourages and facilitates discussion then the true situation may be ignored, becoming the 'elephant in the room' – something unavoidable, impossible to dismiss, but not acknowledged (Griffie *et al.*, 2004).

Griffie *et al.* (2004) goes on to challenge nurses with three key tasks to help prevent this situation arising:

- to create an environment that facilitates communication;
- to enable two-way communication between the patient/family and the health care professionals involved;
- to facilitate communication between the patient and family as and when necessary.

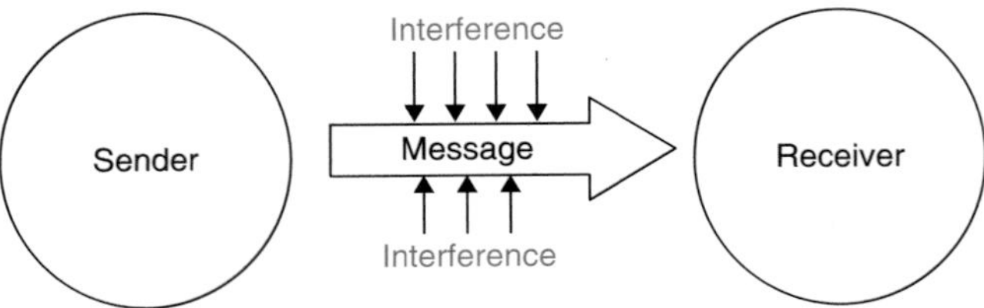

Figure 6.2 Process of communication.

Communication theory

Whilst the literature contains many definitions of communication, ranging from the highly technical to the more human (Bach and Grant, 2010), there is no single definition on which all agree. There are common themes, for example it is a process that involves an exchange of information, ideas and feelings and includes verbal and non-verbal components. The process begins with a sender who encodes the message they want to send. Their own values and beliefs, along with their expectations and their interpretation of the environment all contribute to the way in which the message is encoded and sent. The message has to pass through 'interference' to the recipient, who then decodes it. This decoding process will depend on the receiver's values and beliefs, expectations and their interpretation of the environment. The communication can only be considered successful if the messages sent are interpreted by the receiver with the meaning attributed by the sender. This is often apparent by the recipients response, who on receiving the message becomes a sender and the process is carried out in reverse. This is illustrated in Figure 6.2.

Communication is often divided into three distinct sections – verbal, non-verbal and paralinguistics or paralanguage. Whilst verbal communication relates to the spoken or written word, non-verbal communication refers to body language (Gordon *et al.*, 2006). Hargie and Dickson (2004: p. 44) define non-verbal communication as *all forms of direct communication not exclusively relying on the use of words, written or spoken*. Non-verbal communication is often decisive in conveying information and enabling judgements about others. For example, aspects of our appearance convey our age group, gender, aspects of our personality and can often convey occupation and status.

Hargie and Dickson (2004) identify the following six forms of non-verbal communication:

1. haptics – communication through physical touch;
2. kinesics – communication through body movements;
3. proxemics – when a message is conveyed through perception and use of personal or social space;
4. physical characteristics – conveying information through body shape, size decorations etc.;
5. environmental factors – when messages are carried by features of social surroundings, furniture, décor, lighting etc.;
6. vocalics – communication by means of non-verbal elements of speech, for example, pitch, tone, speed.

Activity 6.3

Consider the forms of non-verbal communication identified by Hargie and Dickson. Try and identify a situation when these might be used in a palliative care setting with a positive and negative outcome. Your list may look like the answers in Table 6.2.

Table 6.2 Forms of non-verbal communication and their use in palliative care.

	Positive	Negative
Haptics - touch	To reassure a distressed patient	When the touch is misinterpreted or inappropriate
Kinesics – body movements	Head nodding to encourage a patient to talk about his concerns	Shrugging shoulders in response to a question
Proxemics – using space	Coming down to the patient's level to talk to them	Standing at the foot of the bed to hold a conversation
Physical characteristics	Wearing a clean uniform, appropriate hair, nails etc.	Appearing untidy, paying little attention to physical appearance
Environmental factors – surroundings	A quiet conversation in a secluded area	Having a conversation in an open, non private space
Vocalics – paralinguistic aspects	Using a soft, gentle slow tone to break bad news	Loud, aggressive tones

---

Paralinguistics is defined as the content-free vocalisations and patterns associated with speech such as voice, pitch, volume, pauses and so on, as well as the 'ahs' and 'ums' which may be spoken (Gordon *et al.*, 2006; Berry, 2007). Each person is an individual with a unique voice which will influence the way paralinguistic communication is delivered (Berry, 2007).

This division between verbal and non-verbal communication is artificial and simplistic. In reality they are intertwined and affect each other in transferring meaning (Hargie and Dickson, 2004). An early study by Mehrabian (1972) suggested that in any interaction 55% of the meaning is conveyed through body language, 38% through the non-verbal aspects of speech and only 7% by the words used. For example, when saying 'I'm pleased to see you' with a smile, in a pleasant voice, accompanied by open body language the recipient is more likely to believe it than if the same words are said in a flat monotone, accompanied by a frown and folded arms. The words maybe the same, but in the second example, more meaning will be given to the things that surround them than the words themselves. When there is a mismatch between the verbal and non-verbal message, it is the latter which is likely to convey the true meaning (Berry, 2007). We are often able to carefully monitor what we say, only allowing the true meaning to 'leak out' through lack of attention to how we are saying it (Hargie and Dickson, 2004).

Palliative care nursing requires us to communicate successfully with patients, families and health care professionals. The ability to achieve this requires us not only to use the correct words and display appropriate non-verbal behaviours and paralinguistics but also to sensitively interpret the communication actions of others (Berry, 2007).

The importance of self-awareness in good communication

If communication is the foundation of good patient care then self-awareness is the foundation for effective communication. Nazarko (2009) estimates that 90% of the information we use to make decisions about people comes from non-verbal sources. Consequently, it is important that through self-awareness we become aware of how we are interpreting the signals of others, and perhaps more importantly, how they might be interpreting the signals we are sending, both consciously and subconsciously.

McCabe and Timmins (2006) argue that self-awareness is a significant tool in the nurse-patient relationship and is indeed a crucial factor in forming a therapeutic relationship. But what is self-awareness? Bach and Grant (2001: p. 147) define self-awareness as:

> our knowledge about ourselves, our motives and how these translate into our behaviours.

This suggests that before we begin to have effective communication with others, we have to be aware of our value and belief systems, how these translate and impact on our motives, thus affecting our behaviours. For example, a staff nurse admits a patient, they do not 'hit it off' and the nurse believes this is because the patient does not like her. This belief leads her to not liking him/her and she avoids caring for him/her. The patient senses this and the nurse overhears him saying to his visitor 'I don't like that nurse much. She's been funny with me ever since I was admitted'. This made the nurse realise how much her behaviour had contributed to the situation.

Activity 6.4

Think of a time when you felt someone misunderstood or misread you. How did it make you feel and how did you react and behave?

Spend some time considering what you might have done or said to contribute to the confusion. Was it what you were saying or maybe your body language, posture or something else? Try to identify what you could do differently to prevent this happening again.

In addition to being self aware, it is important to posses key communication skills in order to communicate effectively with patients and their families.

Key communication skills

Listening

The importance of really listening to patients and families receiving palliative care cannot be over emphasised. Indeed nurses who listen to patients' stories, learn about them and take time to 'just be with them' are perceived by patients as being caring (Betcher, 2010). Listening is a skill that is often taken for granted, because it is something considered as a given, that is, done all the time. In fact, more often than not passive listening occurs, the listener is not really engaged in the process.

Activity 6.5

Think of a time when you felt someone was really listening to you. What was it like? How did you feel? What did your listener do or not do which helped create the sense of being heard?

Active listening has been described as listening with all the senses. It requires us to not only listen to the words being said but also to pay careful attention to the non-verbal messages as well as the tone, pitch, etc. surrounding them. It is hearing what is not being said as well what is. Read the brief exchange between Bill and Sarah in Box 6.1.

Sarah has two choices here. She can take the words at face value, concluding that considering it was Bill's first night in hospital and in a strange bed he had a reasonable night's sleep, leaving the interaction there. Conversely, observing Bill's body language and listening to his tone might make Sarah ask a follow up question. See Box 6.2.

If we fail to hear all that is being said we miss the opportunity of exploring any worries, fears or troublesome symptoms that patients are experiencing. When actively listening, we are really able to engage with patients and gain a far deeper understanding of their experiences.

Strategies for active listening include the following:

- stopping – focussing on the other person and their thoughts and feelings. This requires forgetting about our own concerns and worries, giving full attention to the speaker;
- looking – paying attention to the non-verbal messages, whilst still attending to the spoken word;
- listening – for the essence of the speaker's thoughts whilst trying to gain an overall understanding of what the speaker is trying to communicate, rather than concentrating on the words or terms they use;
- empathy – be empathetic to the feelings of the speaker, remaining calm;
- questioning – to clarify understanding as well as demonstrating interest.

It is important to show the speaker that you are actively listening. This is achieved through a good match between the listener's verbal, non-verbal and paralinguistic communication, for example, appropriate body language, head nodding, encouragement, pace and tone of speech with appropriate re-enforcement, reflection, summary and checking of information.

Box 6.1 Interaction between Bill and Sarah

Consider this interaction between Sarah – the staff nurse and Bill who has just spent his first night in hospital following an admission with increased pain.

Sarah: Morning Bill. How did you sleep last night?
Bill: Not so bad thanks.

Box 6.2 Alternative interaction between Bill and Sarah

Sarah: Morning Bill. How did you sleep last night?
Bill: Not so bad thanks.
Sarah: Not so bad can mean not so good. How much sleep did you actually have last night?
Bill: I suppose in total about an hour and a half.
Sarah: How much did the pain keep you awake?
Bill: Quite a bit really. I settled OK and went off about 11.00. But I woke up with this gnawing pain in my back about 12.30 and couldn't go back off.
Sarah: So what were you thinking about?
Bill: Well ....

Questioning

Being able to ask questions effectively is a core communication skill (Berry, 2007). The purpose of questioning includes opening discussions, gain information, establishing feelings, attitudes and demonstrating interest. There are many types of questions. Spend a moment trying to identify all types of questions you can think of. Your list may include the following types of questions:

- open
- closed
- clarifying
- probing
- leading
- multiple

Open questions are those types of questions to which it is difficult to give a 'yes' or 'no' answer. They allow longer unstructured answers allowing the patient to say how things are in their own words. Open questions begin with one of the following six words:

- who
- what
- where
- when
- why
- how

A note of caution, however, is necessary when using 'Why?' as it carries with it a suggestion of judgement. For example 'Why did you do that?' suggests that something different should have been done. People may well be wrong-footed when faced with a 'why' question and become defensive. Rather than promoting a discussion, it may have the opposite effect and cause the patient to withdraw. It is always worth taking a moment to try and rephrase a 'why' question. For example 'Why didn't you take your MST on time?' could be rephrased as 'What stopped you taking your MST on time?'

Whilst open questions are invaluable to find out more, sometimes they can produce a lot of irrelevant and unwanted material. So consider giving the patient some direction or focus when using open questions. For example, 'How have you been since I last saw you?' or 'What did you have for breakfast today?' might produce far more relevant information than 'How are you?' or 'How's your appetite?'

Closed questions are those which require a 'yes' or 'no' answer, for example, 'can you', 'did you', 'are you', 'would you'. They are useful to obtain a limited amount of factual information. They may, however, result in the patient feeling frustrated as they allow little opportunity for them to express how they feel (Berry, 2007).

The use of closed questions could be considered poor communication, particularly in a speciality where communication is so important. They do have their place, however, and the skill is to know when to use them. They may be particularly useful for patients who have difficulties in formulating the longer answers required for open questions, for example, the cognitively impaired, or a person for whom English is not his/her first language.

Clarifying questions are used to clarify a point or an issue. For example, a person might say 'I feel a bit down today'. But what does this really mean? The meaning therefore need to be checked out and clarified before any response is given. For example, 'A bit down means different things to different people, what does it mean to you?'

Sometimes patients need to be challenged in order to find out more about what they mean. This requires the use of questions which probe that that bit deeper. For example, 'tell me more about ......?' 'what did you think when you heard that ......?' Probing questions are helpful to clarify issues(Hargie and Dickson, 2004).

Leading questions are those which give the recipient a clue as to what the expected answer should be. For example 'You don't want pain killer do you?' or 'You slept well didn't you?' Rhetorical questions on the other hand need no response at all.

Multiple questions are confusing for both the recipient and the questioner. For example, if the patient was asked 'Did you sleep well? What do you want for breakfast? And any pain today?' all in one go, s/he would not know which one to answer first. The chances are patients will answer the question they perceive most important to them, while the questioner may have different priorities.

All questions have a place in communicating with patients who have palliative care needs. The skill is in knowing which type to ask when and to remember that the wrong type of question, if accompanied by inappropriate non-verbal language and paralingusitics, will impede rather than facilitate communication.

Reflecting

In the context of skilled interpersonal communication, reflection is closely associated with active listening (Dickson, 2006). Having heard what has been said, the listener can act like a mirror and reflect back to the speaker the meanings and feelings they have heard. It can involve paraphrasing factual content as well as trying to reflect and understand the feelings identified (Berry, 2007). Some of the functions of reflection are shown in Box 6.3.

Box 6.3 Function of reflection in communication (adapted from Hargie and Dickson, 2004)

- demonstrates an interest in and involvement with the speaker;
- indicates close attention is being paid;
- shows that the listener is trying to understand what is being said;
- checks out the listener's perceptions and understanding;
- helps to facilitate the speaker's understanding and clarity of thought;
- communicates a deep concern for what the speaker considers important;
- places emphasis on the speaker;
- validates the speaker's thoughts and feelings;
- helps the speaker to realise that thoughts can influence behaviours;
- helps the listener to understand reasons and motives underlying patient behaviours.

Look at the interaction in Box 6.4, between Sally (a patient) and Ben (the CNS)

In this interaction, Ben helps Sally face up to the fact that she is frightened about going home. He does this by actively listening to her words and hearing what is being said within them. He reflects back to her those feelings and as he does that, Sally acknowledges their validity.

Reflecting can involve paraphrasing, which means the listener reflects in his/her own words the essential content of what the speaker has just said (Hargie and Dickson, 2004). The emphasis

Box 6.4 Interaction between Sally and Ben

Ben: How did you feel after the ward round when the consultant told you you could go home tomorrow?

Long pause

Sally: To be honest I wasn't too happy about it. I want to go home and be with the children of course I do – it's just that I wasn't expecting it just yet.

Ben: You weren't expecting it just yet?

Sally: No – I thought I would be in at least another week. I just feel as though it's too soon. I've only been on these new pain killers for two days and they are OK now but what if they don't work at home. I mean I do more when I'm there; I want to do more – you know look after the children and Tom and what if the pain comes back. I just couldn't face all that pain again.

Ben: I think what you are telling me is that you feel safe here and you are frightened of going home. You think the pain may come back because you won't be able to care for your family the way you want to

Long pause

Sally: Yes you're right. I am scared – terrified in fact.

is on the factual content of what has been said, and according to Hargie and Dickson (2004) there are three important elements to the paraphrase which are as follows:

1. it must be couched in the speakers own words;
2. it should contain the essential component of the message;
3. it primarily reflects factual information.

Summarising

This is a really important communication skill to develop as it has a number of uses. First, it allows both parties the opportunity to agree on what has been discussed. Second, it can help to convey that the listener has understood what has been said, giving the speaker the opportunity to correct any errors. Third, a summary can act as a 'breathing space' providing the opportunity to reflect on what has been said and identify where the conversation needs to go next.

Effective communication is not only dependent on the skills of the nurse but there are also situations which enhance or impede communication. It is important to be aware of the enablers of and barriers to good communication.

Enablers of and barriers to good communication

In their systematic review of communication in end-of-life care, Parker *et al.* (2007) concluded that health care professionals should not make assumptions about the information needs of patients and their carers as everyone is an individual with needs that are different and likely to change at various stages of the illness. Patients and carers wanted clear information, delivered in small jargon free chunks with empathy, care, compassion and honesty balanced with sensitivity and hope (Parker *et al.*, 2007). The challenge is to achieve this.

If we consider the diagram in Figure 6.2, it is clear that enablers of effective communication can be anything that

- allows the sender to recognise an appropriate message and encode effectively;
- minimises the interference during transit;
- allows the recipient to receive the message and decode it accurately.

Conversely, barriers to effective communication can be anything that hinders this process.

Activity 6.6

Consider the communication diagram in Figure 6.2.

Spend some time thinking about the factors which can influence the process.

Think about those factors which may influence the way the sender encodes the message.

Consider those factors which may influence the way in which the receiver decodes the message.

Consider those factors which might interfere with the message.

Your ideas may be similar to those represented in Figure 6.3.

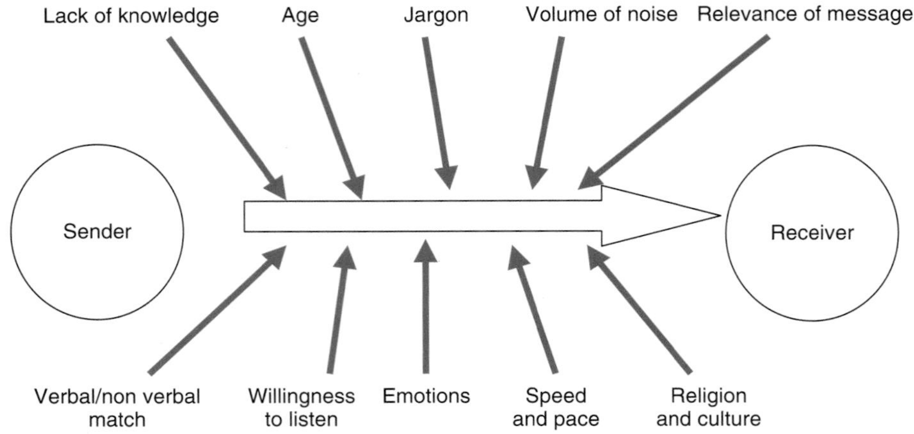

Figure 6.3 Influences on the communication process.

Influencing factors

a. Age

As we age, senses diminish. Whilst 60% of 70-year-olds will have some degree of hearing loss, the figures rises to 90% in people aged 90 (Nazarko, 2009). Older people also need 60% more light than younger people; poorly lit rooms may inhibit their ability to communicate, specifically in interpreting non-verbal signals correctly.

Whilst age itself has challenges in communication, age differences also have a considerable impact. Different generations often seem to speak different languages as new words enter the vocabulary whilst others leave. We need to consider this factor when talking to patients from a different generation.

b. Disease

All patients are individuals and therefore their reactions to their illness will also be unique. Communication needs may well change as the illness progresses, particularly when a patient living with a chronic disease such as severe heart failure or multiple sclerosis enters the final stages of their illness.

Some diseases such as dementia or a brain tumour affect cognitive functioning; the person's ability to understand is affected, others such as Parkinson's Disease and Motor Neurone Disease affect motor ability. Whilst the former group have difficulties comprehending the message, the latter have difficulties in sending one.

The likely prognosis or disease trajectory may well affect the communication process. Some life-limiting illnesses have a more easily estimated prognosis than others. For example, 50% of patients admitted to hospital with an acute exacerbation of heart failure today will be dead in six months – the problem is that there is nothing to identify to which half any particular patient belongs. When the future is uncertain it may be more difficult to initiate conversations relating to future care planning.

c. Environment

The environment affects the outcome of a communication interaction. Background noise, interruptions, room temperature and distractions can all negatively affect an interaction. When the patient is in the hospital we can sometimes have more control over the environment than when the patient is at home. Wherever possible, it is good practice to choose a quite room free from distractions. Some patients, however, might be more comfortable talking with the noise from television in the background. The challenge there for the nurse is to stop becoming distracted by a sound commentary.

Positioning is an important consideration when talking with patients. It is important for the listener and speaker to be at the same level where possible and this may require the nurse to sit on the floor. Egan (1998) recommends the acronym SOLER as a way of helping to remember key behaviours that facilitate active listening and communication. The meaning is as follows:

- **S** sit squarely in relation to the patient
- **O** adopt an open position with the body
- **L** lean slightly forward towards the patient
- **E** engage in eye contact
- **R** relax, encouraging the patient to relax.

Whilst this can be helpful, it is important to remember that having someone sitting squarely in front of you can, in certain circumstances, be uncomfortable as it makes breaking eye contact very difficult. When engaged in conversation, the speaker tends to establish eye contact with the listener at the start, breaking it as their input develops to re-establish just before they conclude, thus signalling to the listener that it is nearly their turn to contribute. Sitting squarely in front of someone can make this process more difficult as breaking eye contact requires the speaker to make a deliberate head movement.

A solution is to sit more off-centre so that both speakers as they take turns in talking can break eye contact very comfortably by just looking over the listener's shoulder. By bringing their eyes back eye contact can simply be re-established.

Activity 6.7

Consider the seating arrangements shown in Figure 6.4. The first reflects SOLER whilst the second illustrates the more off-centre approach.

Try having a conversation with a friend using both of these positions. In which position did you find most comfortable and helpful to converse? What were the advantages and disadvantages of both?

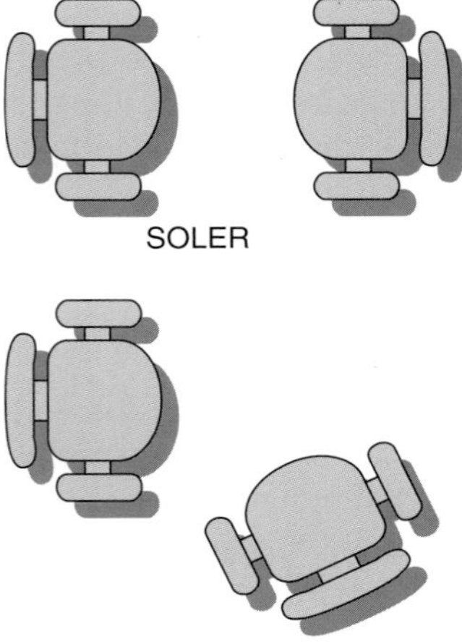

Figure 6.4 Seating arrangements.

d. Language

When the speaker and listener speak different languages, the potential for things to go wrong is huge. When thinking of different languages, it is easy to assume that this occurs only when the participants are from different countries or cultures. This is a very limited view. The fact that different ages speak different 'languages' has already been mentioned, but we also need to recognise that different areas of the United Kingdom have different dialects and use words which can make it sound as though they speak a different language. It is also true that health care professionals often use their own language, littered with jargon with which the lay person may not be familiar.

e. Nurse

Nurses must be willing to listen and engage with the other person. They must ensure that their verbal and non-verbal language match and the message they want to send is relevant to the listener. There is also a need for them to be aware of how they are impacting on the interaction.

Communicating with groups who have particular needs

Communicating with any patient who has palliative care needs is challenging as well as rewarding. Each patient is an individual with a unique set of circumstances and history. We need to use communication skills effectively in order to deliver good palliative care to each person. Some groups of patients, however, have specific challenges. These include those with mental health issues, learning disabilities, those living with dementia, those from different ethnic or cultural backgrounds and those whose first language is not English.

Whilst the skills needed maybe very similar, the way they are used may require adapting. The nurse may also have to increase her knowledge for a specific patient. For example, rules regarding eye contact differ across cultures and what might be normal within the British culture may be considered rude and offensive in others. In Western cultures we have a far more open approach to sharing diagnosis and prognosis than Eastern cultures. If English is not spoken or not spoken well, it may be necessary to employ the services of an interpreter. For convenience this is often a family member who carries with him/her a whole host of concerns and issues. For example, there is no way of knowing if the communication of either party is being translated accurately. It is good practice to use the interpreters appointed by the hospital wherever possible. Those who have difficulty communicating because of the effects of the disease that impair cognitive abilities may need a very personalised approach and we need to seek the help of their usual carers, lay or professional, to help interpret what they mean. For example, pain may often be expressed as changes in behaviour or vocalisations.

Conclusion

Recognising the importance of communication in palliative care can improve our abilities to care for this group of patients. Understanding basic communication theory can improve our practice as we develop our skills. We must recognise the way we impact on communication through increasing self-awareness. Key communication skills, once mastered, can be transferred to various situations. It is important to recognise that what may be a barrier to effective communication in one setting may enable it in another. Finally, recognising that everyone is an individual with their own needs and concerns will help us communicate with those who have particular needs.

Glossary

Active listening Listening with all the senses; fully engaged in the process.

Body language Movements of the hands, legs, gestures, eye contact and facial expressions.

Clarifying questions Used to elicit more information.

Closed questions Can be answered by a simple 'yes' or 'no'.

Communication The meaningful exchange of information between two or more people.

Haptics Communication through physical touch, a component of non-verbal communication.

Kinesics Communication through body movements; a component of non-verbal communication.

Leading questions The recipient receives a clue as to the expected answer.

Multiple questions The recipient receives several questions to answer at the same time.

Non-verbal communication	Conveying information in the form of wordless cues.
Open questions	Questions to which it is difficult to give a simple 'yes' or 'no' answer.
Probing questions	Seek to delve more deeply into an issue.
Passive listening	Occurs when the listener is not completely engaged in the process.
Paralinguistics	The content free vocalisations and patterns associated with speech.
Paraphrasing	Reflect on what has been said in the listener's words.
Patient-centred care	Care which puts the patient at the centre.
Proxemics	When a message is conveyed through perception and use of personal space; a component of non-verbal communication.
Reflecting	In communication, this is linked to active listening and paraphrasing to the speaker the feelings and words they have used.
Rhetorical questions	Do not need an answer.
Self-awareness	The capacity for introspection and the ability to recognise oneself as an individual separate from the environment and others.
SOLER	An acronym for sitting squarely; open posture; lean inwards; eye contact; relax.
Summarising	Drawing together what has been said.
Therapeutic relationship	The relationship between a nurse and patient where both engage with each other in the hope of bringing about a positive change for the patient.
Verbal communication	Messages conveyed through words which may be spoken or written.
Vocalics	Non-verbal elements of speech, such as pitch, tone, speed.

References

Bach, S. and Grant, A. (2010) *Communication and Interpersonal Skills in Nursing* 2nd edn. Exeter: Learning Matters Ltd.

Berry, D. (2007) *Health Communication Theory and Practice* Maidenhead: Open University Press.

Betcher, D.K. (2010) Elephant in the room project: improving caring efficacy through effective and compassionate communication with palliative care patients. *MEDSUR Nursing.* 19 (2): 101–105.

Dickson, D. (2006) Reflecting In Hargie, O. (ed) *The Handbook of Communication Skills.* 3rd edn, London: Routledge Chapter 6.

Egan, G. (1998) *The Skilled Helper.* London: Brooks Cole.

Gordon, R.A., Druckman, D., Rozelle, R.M. and Baxter, J.C. (2006) Non-verbal behaviour as communication: approaches, issues and research In Hargie, O. (ed) *The Handbook of Communication Skills* 3rd edn. London: Routledge Chapter 3.

Griffie, J., Nelson-Martin, P. and Muchka, S. (2004) Acknowledging the 'Elephant': Communication in Palliative Care. *American Journal of Nursing* 104 (1): 48–57.

Hargie, O. and Dickson, D. (2004) *Skilled Interpersonal Communication Research Theory and Practice* 4th edn. East Sussex: Routledge.

McCabe, C. and Timmins, F. (2006) *Communication Skills for Nursing Practice.* London: Palgrave Macmillan.

Mehrabian, A. (1972). *Nonverbal communication.* Chicago, IL: Aldine-Atherton.

Nazarko, L. (2009) Advanced communication skills. *Journal of Healthcare Assistants.* 3 (9): 449–452.

Parker, S.M., Clayton, J.M., Hancock, K., Walder, S., Butow, P. N., Carrick, S., Currow, D., Ghersi, D., Glare, P., Hagerty, R. and Tattersill, M.H.N. (2007) A systematic review of prognostic/end-of-life communication with adults in the advanced stages of a life-limiting illness: patient/caregiver preferences for the content, style and timing of information. *Journal of Pain and Symptom Management.* 34 (1): 81–93.

Smith, B. and Field, L. (2011) *Nursing Care An essential Guide for Nurses and Healthcare Workers in Primary and Secondary Care* 2nd edn. Harlow: Pearson Education Limited.

7

Pain management and nursing care

Introduction

According to the WHO (2014) definition of palliative care, it is clear that impeccable assessment of all symptoms, including pain, is vital to ensure accurate diagnosis and appropriate management. This chapter focuses on assessment and nursing and medical management of pain for patients receiving palliative care.

Learning outcomes

By the end of this chapter you will be able to

- recognise the importance of an impeccable assessment in pain management;
- discuss the use of pain assessment tools;
- understand the principles of pain management;
- discuss the nurse's role in managing pain.

Fundamentals of Palliative Care for Student Nurses, First Edition. Megan Rosser and Helen C. Walsh.

Companion website: www.wiley.com/go/rosser_walsh/fundamentals_of_palliative_care

Pain

What is pain?

As early as 1968 a nurse offered the following definition of pain:

> Pain is what the person says it is and exists whenever he or she says it does
>
> *McCaffery, 1968*

This definition highlights the subjective nature of pain and continues to be a cornerstone of optimal pain management. If we do not listen to the patient and understand their perceptions of their pain we will never succeed in understanding the patient's pain experience.

Having established that the patient is best placed to describe their pain experience it is important to appreciate that pain is a complex experience made up of both physical and psychological components. A more clinical definition of pain articulates the complexity of the pain experience:

> An unpleasant sensory and emotional experience associated with actual or potential tissue damage, or described in terms of such damage
>
> *International Association for the Study of Pain (2012)*

Pathophysiology of pain

The pathophysiology of pain is explained in another book in this series (Wheeldon, 2009); however, it is important to know what causes pain and what different types of pain people experience. Pain results from the activation of nociceptors (pain receptors) by actual or potential tissue damage, which provokes the release of pain producing chemicals such as bradykinin, substance P and prostaglandins as part of the inflammatory response. These chemicals stimulate nociceptive neurons and the impulses from these neurons are carried through the ascending pathway in the spinothalamic tract to the thalamus and cortex. The brain interprets the impulses as pain in the thalamus and through more complicated processing in the cortex is able to determine the location of the pain and interprets both the physical and emotional components of the pain (Harlos and MacDonald, 2005). This is represented in Figure 7.1.

Causes of pain

Patients receiving palliative care are most likely to be experiencing chronic pain that has occurred as a result of:

- their disease – altered muscle tone/muscle spasm, tumour pressure;
- their disease treatment – drugs, therapies, chemo/radiotherapy;
- debility – stiffness, pressure ulcers, comorbidity.

Pain can be largely divided into two main types – nociceptive and neuropathic, see Figure 7.2

Types of pain

Pain can be either acute or chronic; whilst acute pain is temporary with a foreseeable end and serves as a warning of injury or disease, chronic pain serves no such purpose. Chronic pain is

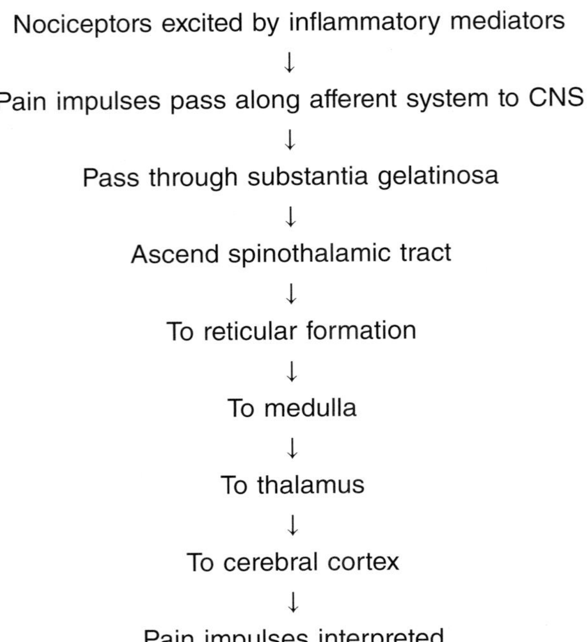

Figure 7.1 The pain pathway.

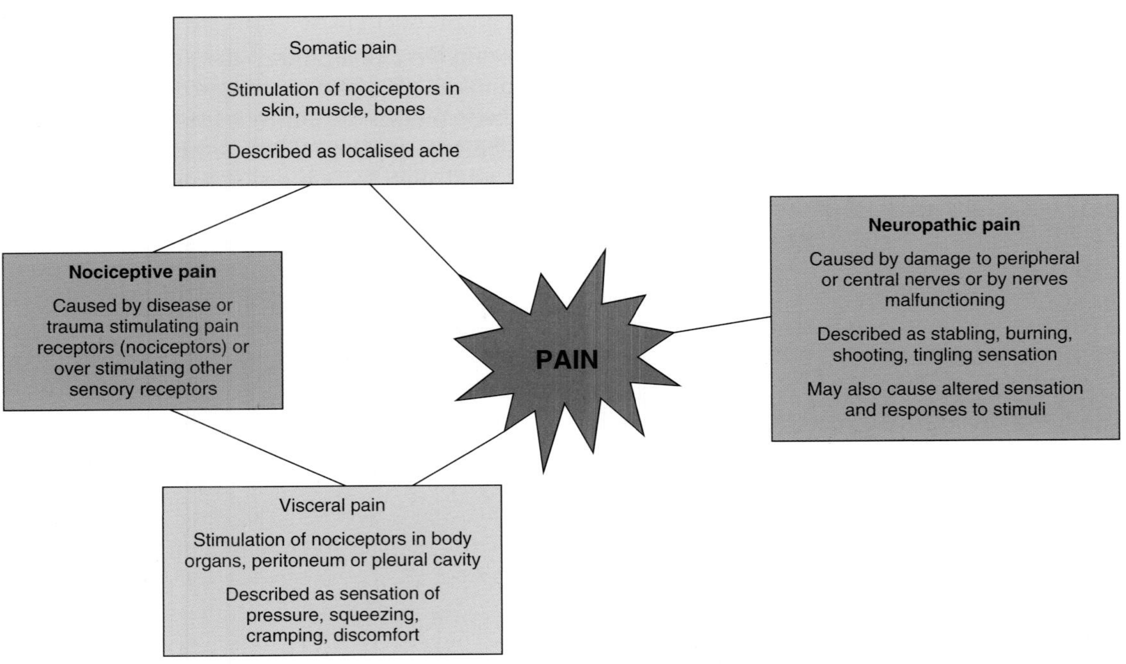

Figure 7.2 Types of pain.

Fact Box 7.1

Incidence of pain for different patient groups – Percentage of patients experiencing pain

Heart failure	Up to 78%
COPD	70%
CKD	47%
Stroke	Up to 74%
MS	57–65%
MND	up to 73%
Cancer	25% of patients have pain at diagnosis, 75% will experience pain during their illness 25% will not- this is an important figure because most people associate diagnosis of cancer with pain

(Salt, 2003; Oliver *et al.*, 2007; Dean, 2008, South West London Cardiac Network, 2009; Russon and Mooney, 2010; Lalkhen *et al.*, 2012; National Stroke Association, 2012)

persistent and reminds people of their disease. Chronic pain is a common problem for many people receiving palliative care as shown in Fact Box 7.1 above.

Pain assessment

To be able to manage pain effectively it is vital to undertake a comprehensive, holistic assessment. The assessment enables a member of the team to identify the cause of that pain and the most appropriate treatment. Some pains are more complex than others and will require input from the members of the specialist palliative care team. The more straightforward pains can be managed effectively by knowledgeable practitioners in any health care setting. There are well-established principles of pain assessment and management which, if adhered to, will result in good pain control for the vast majority of patients.

The first stage in successful management of pain is comprehensive assessment. A good pain assessment will be based on the patient's self report of their pain experience. The assessing nurse needs to be a good communicator, using listening and observation skills in particular. Asking the patient about their pain has a positive impact on most patients; it makes them feel listened to. This may be the first time that a patient's pain has really been acknowledged and that in itself can have a positive effect for the patient. If the assessment is patient-led there will be minimal room for professional interpretation or judgement, which might result in the patient's pain being underestimated and consequently undertreated.

A comprehensive pain assessment will enable nurses to identify the nature of the pain; this helps identify the likely cause of the pain and how it would be managed best. There are a number of different types of pain, with many different causes and if the cause of the pain is not identified accurately, it will not be possible for the correct drugs to be prescribed to relieve that pain.

Activity 7.1

Think of the things you would ask a patient if you wanted to know more about their pain, list your questions and compare to those in Figure 7.3.

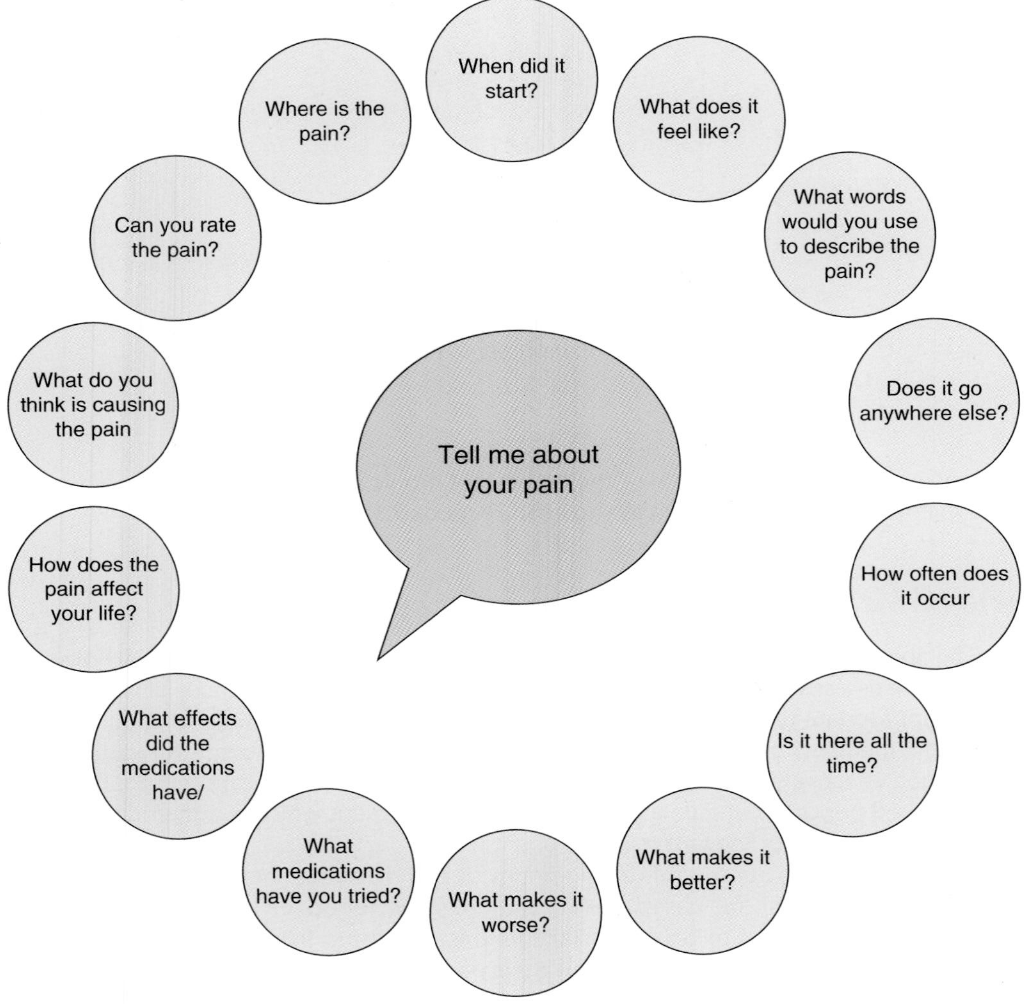

Figure 7.3 Questions to ask during a pain assessment.

Patients' description will often indicate the type of pain they are experiencing, for example, reports of continuous pain are suggestive of visceral/soft tissue pain, pain on movement may suggest bone pain, while stabbing/burning pain characteristics may be associated with nerve pain. In addition to asking a patient these questions, it is also important to think about whether there might be other factors that make him/her more susceptible to pain or that makes him/her more able to bear pain. This will include thinking about their individual pain threshold.

Pain thresholds

The pain threshold is the level at which someone starts to feel pain; we all have different pain thresholds and would experience a painful stimulus differently from everyone else in nature and intensity.

Activity 7.2

Think of things that might make you feel pain more easily (i.e. lower your pain threshold) or might stop you feeling pain (i.e. raise your pain threshold) Compare your answers to those in Figure 7.4.

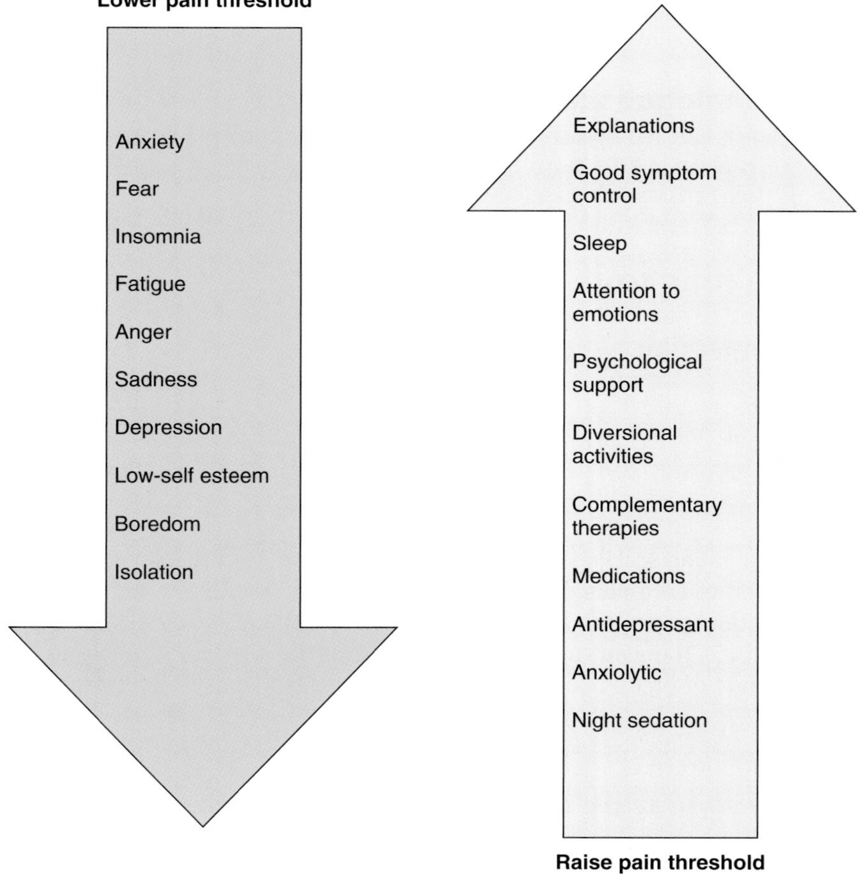

Figure 7.4 Factors influencing pain thresholds.

Pain assessment tools

The questions in Figure 7.2 form part of the formal pain assessment. There are a number of pain assessment tools that are used to incorporate and supplement the information gained by questioning patients. These range from simple rating scales to long, multi-faceted pain assessment tools. You are probably most familiar with the simple rating scales and may even use them as part of your NEWS assessment of patients. The longer, multi-faceted tools are used more often by specialist palliative care teams who are working with patients experiencing complex pains, which are more difficult to manage.

Rating scales include:

The numerical rating scale (NRS):

No pain									Worst pain imaginable
0	1	2	3	4	5	6	7	8	9	10

A 10 cm line is divided into 1 cm notches to enable the patient to attach a numerical score to their pain. Patients are asked to allocate a score to the intensity of pain that they are feeling.

The visual analogue scale (VAS):

A 10 cm long line is labelled at each end with opposite intensities of pain; patients are asked to identify the point along the line which reflects the intensity of the pain they are experiencing.

No pain ______________________________________ Worst pain Imaginable

The verbal rating score (VRS):

Patients are asked to rate their pain in association with a list of words that describe pain increasing in intensity:

0 no pain
1 mild pain
2 moderate pain
3 severe pain

While all three rating scales have been found to be valid and reliable, patients dislike the VAS finding it hardest to complete; the VRS is the simplest to complete but patients like the NRS best for it provides data about the changing nature of the intensity of their pain (Williamson and Hoggart, 2005). It may also follow that the NRS is the easiest for nurses to use in order to evaluate the effect of pharmacological and non-pharmacological interventions.

Body charts

Body charts are also useful tools in pain assessment. Use of a body chart enables the patient to indicate where their pain is. It is worth noting that some patients will have more than one pain and use of the body chart helps nurses to understand which pain the patient is talking about during different points in the assessment. Most patients will be capable of filling in their own body charts and may like to be actively involved in their pain assessment.

Other pain assessment tools

When patients have complex pains that require referral to the specialist palliative care team, practitioners will undertake a more in depth pain assessment using a pain assessment tool such as the Brief Pain Inventory or the McGill Pain Questionnaire (Chapman 2012). These tools explore the patient's pain experience in far greater depth, enabling the team to get to the bottom of the likely cause of the pain.

Barriers to pain assessment

Impeccable pain assessment is fundamental to optimal pain management; however, this does not always occur. There are barriers that arise on the part of either the nurse or the patient and this need to be overcome to ensure adequate information is obtained to enable correct diagnosis of the cause of pain. Some nurses lack the knowledge and skills required to carry out an appropriate pain assessment; failing to focus on the holistic nature of the pain, they may not even know to use a formal pain assessment tool. Nurses need to use their communication skills to establish a therapeutic relationship with the patient so that he/she feels safe to talk about his/her pain. Nurses may question the validity of the patients self reporting; some put their own judgement on a patient's pain experience. This judgement causes the nurse to over or underestimate the patient's pain and is often influenced by his/her own experiences of pain. The patient's self report is disregarded and the nurse's own impression is presented. In worst cases, the patient's self report is just not believed, because they 'don't look in pain' or 'they are moving around' or 'their obs are fine'. Nurses may lack knowledge about chronic pain syndromes that patients with chronic illnesses experience; therefore, the information gained from a pain assessment may not be correctly interpreted by the nurse so an incorrect diagnosis is made. It must be accepted that the person best placed to assess the pain accurately is the patient.

Patients, however, may be unwilling to report pain; this occurs for a number of reasons. Some patients believe that pain is part of their illness and something they have to put up with. Some people are just stoical by nature while others do not like to bother nurses or doctors so they suffer in silence. Some patients associate pain with progression of their disease so keep silent, while some patients fear that if they say their pain is getting worse they may be prescribed stronger drugs; therefore, they prefer to keep quiet. Once a therapeutic relationship has been established, the nurse must spend time listening to the patient and encouraging him/her to speak openly about his/her pain.

There are particular groups of patients who may find it challenging to communicate their pain to nurses. These include patients who have cognitive problems or communication problems. Pain assessment becomes more complex and different approaches of assessment are needed for these patients. It is acknowledged that pain is under-recognised in these patient groups (McAuliffe *et al.*, 2008); therefore, it is important that particular care is taken when trying to assess pain in these vulnerable groups. For instance, people with dementia are likely only to be able to relate to pain experienced in the present, their diminished recall makes it difficult to report pain experienced previously. Simpler assessment tools may be necessary to help people with dementia, learning difficulties and other cognitive problems. These simpler tools include smiley faces, coloured scales, and pictures (Chatterjee, 2012). Where patients' cognitive functioning is severely impaired, there is a tendency of carers to rely on observation of mood and behaviour for signs of pain. These observations can be used as part of pain assessment using the Abbey pain scale (Abbey *et al.*, 2004). Nurses need to know their patients well so that they can differentiate between normal and abnormal behaviours for each of their patients.

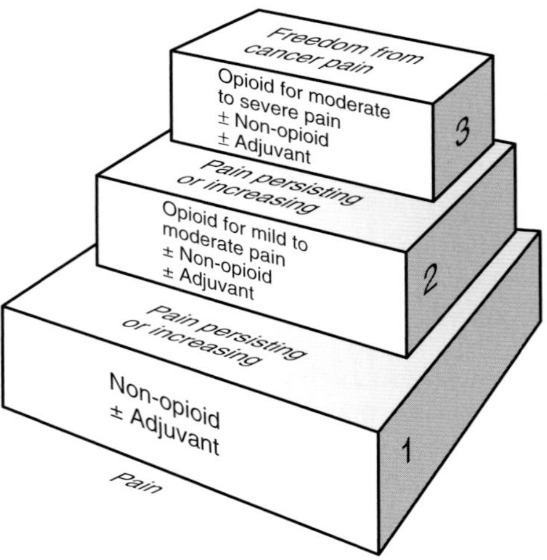

Figure 7.5 World Health Organisation analgesic ladder.

Principles of pain management

Once the type of pain has been identified there are central principles that need to be adhered to, regardless of the medications used to treat the pain. These include the following:

- medication:
  - by mouth, if possible;
  - by the clock, analgesia must be given regularly, not on a PRN basis;
  - by the ladder (see Figure 7.5).
- individual prescribing
- continual review
- attend to pain thresholds
- realistic aims.

Prescribing according to the WHO ladder

While there have been some recent criticisms of the WHO analgesic ladder, it is still accepted as the cornerstone for guiding prescribing in palliative care (Vargas-Schaffer, 2010). For patients who present with mild to moderate pain, WHO recommends that prescribing starts with a non-opioid such as

- aspirin;
- a non-steroidal anti-inflammatory drug (NSAIDs) such as ibuprofen;
- paracetamol.

All of these drugs have anti-inflammatory properties and inhibit prostaglandin synthesis, thus reducing stimulation of the nociceptors. They are particularly useful in controlling pain from bone or soft tissue damage. Adjuvant analgesics (discussed later) may be prescribed depending on the pain type.

If the pain persists or worsens, or if patients report moderate or severe pain at the first assessment, then move on to step 2, which recommend the prescription of weak opioids. These include the codeine-based drugs such as co-codamol, and co-dydramol and the non-codeine based tramadol. When patients take codeine based drugs the codeine is converted into morphine in the liver for analgesic effect.

Weak opioids can be prescribed with NSAIDs, adjuvant analgesics and also paracetamol (if the weak opioid does not contain paracetamol). All these analgesics affect the pain pathways in different ways so are useful in combination. It is important that the medications are prescribed to their maximum dose before progressing to the final step. If the patient's pain does not respond, then it is necessary to progress to step 3. A common mistake is to switch from one weak opioid to another. This will not work; if one weak opioid prescribed at maximum dosage does not control the pain then another one will not either.

Step 3 advocates the use of strong opioids, the most common being morphine. This is the step that you may see people hesitating at; doctors may be reluctant to prescribe morphine for a number of reasons and some patients are reluctant to take it. It is acknowledged that strong opioids, especially morphine, are the main treatment choice for management of pain in advanced progressive disease (NICE, 2012). Reluctance from the doctor or the patient may relate to anxieties about

- perceived as the last resort;
- side effects;
- addiction;
- tolerance – starting too early – will not be effective later;
- perceptions of impending death.

It is important to prescribe analgesia according to the level of pain the patient is experiencing as opposed to the stage of disease that the professionals feel the patient has reached. It is completely appropriate to prescribe morphine early on in the disease process if the severity of the patient's pain requires that level of analgesia.

It is also important to address any concerns that your patient might have about taking morphine so that they take the medication as prescribed. When titrated appropriately against the patient's pain, strong opioids will be effective on most pain types. If patients do not take their medication as prescribed the analgesic effect will be minimal. Patients will think the drug did not work and may lose faith in the professionals looking after them. There is a variety of strong opioids and a variety of routes through which they may be given. You will probably be most familiar with morphine or diamorphine but may well have come across patients taking fentanyl and oxycodone.

Morphine

Morphine can be given as oral immediate release or oral sustained release. NICE (2012) recommend a starting dose of 20–30 mg daily in the preparation that patient prefers. It is important to have immediate release morphine available for rescue doses while the doses are being titrated to the patient's pain. (The rescue dose is 1/6 of the total amount of morphine taken in 24 h). Patients must be reviewed regularly when starting morphine to monitor their response. If patients have impaired liver or renal function, it is recommended that a specialist palliative care practitioner is involved in prescribing strong opioids (NICE, 2012).

Administering PRN doses

As well as analgesics that are prescribed on a regular basis, it is important to have analgesia written up on the PRN side in case the patient experiences pain in between the regular doses of analgesia. Once the patient's analgesic regime has been established the PRN dose for any pain experienced is 1/6 of the total 24-h dose of morphine and is given as immediate release morphine. PRN doses can be given as often as required but a patient requiring frequent PRN doses needs review as the current analgesic regime would appear not to be working.

If a patient is receiving **60 mg MST BD**
The total 24 h dose is **120 mg**
The PRN dose will be 120/6 = **20 mg** oromorph

Side effects of commonly used analgesic drugs

Although analgesics are very effective, most of the drugs advocated for palliative care have side effects. It is good practice to be aware of these so you can advise patients of possible side effects and inform colleagues if patients experience adverse reactions to any of their prescribed drugs.

Paracetamol

Side effects from paracetamol, when taken correctly, are rare. However, paracetamol is extremely toxic to the liver if too many are taken. It is very important then to ensure that patients are not taking paracetamol as well as weak opioids combined with paracetamol.

Aspirin

The most common side effects of aspirin are associated with irritation of the gastro-intestinal tract such as indigestion, nausea and in some cases gastric bleeding. These side effects can generally be prevented by taking aspirin with or after food.

NSAIDS

Because of their effect on prostaglandins, NSAIDS can also precipitate a number of adverse effects including broncho-spasm in asthmatics and, therfore, should be used with caution in this patient group. They can also cause gastric irritation, nausea, vomiting or diarrhoea and may compromise renal function, especially in the elderly. Aspirin and NSAIDS can also inhibit platelet function so extra care needs to be taken if patients are on anticoagulants.

Opioids

Opioids have a number of side effects and it is important that the patient is made aware of these and that the common side effects of constipation, temporary nausea or vomiting and sedation are anticipated.

Constipation occurs because morphine slows down gastric motility, therefore patients commencing morphine need to be prescribed softener and stimulant laxatives. Every time the morphine is increased the dose of laxative must also be reviewed.

Patients may experience temporary nausea when starting morphine because of irritation of the chemoreceptor trigger zone. This can be prevented by prescribing an anti-emetic for the first few days.

Sedation is common when starting or increasing morphine, but is only temporary.

Less common side effects include urinary retention, a dry mouth, sweating and itching.

Although it is known that ordinarily morphine causes respiratory depression (Pattison, 2008), it has long been acknowledged that pain antagonises the respiratory depression associated with morphine, thus maintaining normal respiratory function (International Association for the Study of Pain, 1997). It is, therefore, vital to ensure that the dose of morphine is correctly titrated against the patient's level of pain to ensure that optimal pain relief is achieved without respiratory depression (Estfan *et al.*, 2007). If patients are given too much morphine then respiratory depression will occur.

Some patients may get immense pain relief from morphine but find the side effects unbearable; these patients may be prescribed other strong opioid. For example fentanyl may be given via a transdermal patch. Fentanyl is less constipating and less sedating so is better tolerated. The transdermal route provides a controlled release of fentanyl into the blood via the skin. The patch needs changing every 3 days.

Adjuvant analgesics

While you would not be expected to be advising about these drugs, it is useful for you to know about them to understand a patient's medication history and recommendations that the specialist palliative care team might make for the patients they see. Adjuvant drugs (or co-analgesics) are drugs that were first developed for indications other than pain relief and were later found to have pain relieving properties for specific pains. As indicated in the WHO ladder, they are often added to drug regimes to manage pain that does not respond to the common analgesics such as morphine. Commonly used adjuvant analgesics are listed in Box 7.1.

Anticonvulsants and antidepressants are often used for neuropathic pain, which is particularly difficult to manage. They do have side effects and can also take a couple of weeks before the analgesic effect is felt by the patient.

Anxiolytics can be used to reduce pain from muscle spasm and may also help to relieve muscle tension which is associated with some chronic pain conditions.

Antispasmodics are also used to reduce muscle spasm and spasticity.

Corticosteroids are used to reduce oedema that surrounds tumours and relieve pressure symptoms on adjacent nerves or tissues. They are particularly useful in compression pains such as those caused by bone pain, increased intracranial pressure, nerve pain, liver capsule pain and rectal or pelvic pain. When using steroids for pain control, it is usual to prescribe

Box 7.1 Commonly used adjuvant analgesics

Anticonvulsants	carbamazepine, phenytoin, sodium valproate, gabepentin
Antidepressants	amitriptyline
Anxiolytics	diazepam
Antispasmodics	baclofen
Corticosteroids	dexamethasone, prednisolone

the highest dose and once pain relief occurs the dose is gradually reduced (Hall, 2010). Corticosteroids have a number of side effects and again the patient must be advised about these. These include thrush, oedema, weight gain, cushingnoid appearance, gastric ulceration, neuropsychological effects such as insomnia, restlessness, psychosis, diabetes, myopathy and increased appetite.

When patients are on adjuvant analgesics, it is important that they know why they have been prescribed them. If patients are started on any of these drugs while in your care you may have a place in advising them that the drugs are part of their pain control regime. Patients might read the patient information leaflet in the box once they have been discharged or when the community nurse has gone, and if they have been prescribed an antidepressant or an anticonvulscent they might be worried that there is something else wrong with them and people are withholding information. This provokes unnecessary anxiety and also threatens the trust that is so important within a therapeutic relationship. A little time taken to explain things to the patient and to check out their understanding can prevent these problems.

Palliative radio/chemo therapy for pain management

A patient with cancer may receive palliative radio or chemotherapy as part of his/her pain management regime. Treatment can be used to shrink tumours, thus relieving pain arising from tumour pressure. Palliative radiotherapy is particularly effective in relieving the pain from bone metastases and is generally given as one or two treatments.

Non-pharmacological approaches to pain relief

To achieve optimal pain control it is often helpful to combine pharmacological and non-pharmacological pain management strategies. It is important that any treatment plan is discussed with the patient to ensure that it is acceptable to them. Non-pharmacological interventions can reduce pain and the need for medication, improve patient's mood, instil a sense of well-being, reduce stress, improve functionality and provide the patient with a greater sense of control (Hart, 2008). Most of these will, in turn, increase the pain threshold. Bruckenthal (2010) suggests that non-pharmacological interventions can be divided into the following therapies.

- biological therapies including dietary supplements such as glucosamine, chondroitin (for joint pain) and vitamins. There is some evidence, including a Cochrane review, to suggest efficacy.
- mind-body medicine may provide distraction from the pain or introduce the patient to new ways of dealing with the pain. This group includes prayer, relaxation, guided imagery, meditation, creative therapies, hypnosis and cognitive behavioural therapies. The evidence base suggests that all these are safe practices and may impact positively on patient well being but the impact on pain varies.
- manipulative and body-based practice including physiotherapy, occupational therapy, osteopathy, chiropractic techniques, massage and acupuncture. Help with movement, positioning and flexibility may help alleviate some of the pain. The evidence base for analgesic effects of acupuncture for certain conditions are growing. It is important that all of these therapies are provided by trained practitioners.
- energy medicine including therapeutic touch, reiki and healing touch. The evidence base for these activities is very limited and larger scale studies need to be carried out before any conclusion can be drawn.

Despite combining drugs and therapeutic interventions, there are a number of reasons that pain control is unsuccessful in palliative care. The main reasons are listed below.

- belief that pain is inevitable as chronic diseases progress;
  - health care professionals do not persist with pain management;
  - patients do not mention it to the nurse or doctor;
- pain assessment is incomplete or inaccurate, so it is not possible to identify the true cause of the patient's pain. Therefore, the patient does not receive the most appropriate analgesics;
- insufficient attention may be given to raising the patient's pain threshold where possible;
- the psycho-social components of the patient's pain are not attended to;
- health care professionals may not have the knowledge to prescribe appropriately and may be reluctant to refer to specialist palliative care teams;
- if the patient's pain is not reviewed regularly then necessary changes to medication are not made, therefore, pain control remains sub-optimal.

Conclusion

A comprehensive pain assessment is key to effective management of patient's pain. Assessment must be holistic, taking into account physical, psychological, spiritual and emotional aspects of the patient's experience. Pain is a highly subjective experience; therefore, the patient must be central to the assessment; professionals must not make their own judgements. Once the nature and cause of the pain have been identified the appropriate analgesia or adjuvant analgesia can be prescribed at the correct dosage. Many analgesics cause side effects so it is important for nurses to be familiar with the commonly occurring side effects so they can observe their patients and also educate their patients and families.

Glossary

Acute pain — Sudden onset, temporary pain which serves as warning of illness or injury

Adjuvant analgesia — Drugs whose primary indication is not pain relief but have been proven to have analgesic properties

Anticonvulsant — Drugs primarily used to control epileptic seizures

Antidepressant — Drugs used primarily for treatment of depression and other psychological symptoms such as anxiety

Anxiolytic — Drugs used primarily to relieve anxiety

Bradykinin — Powerful inflammatory mediator released from plasma from damaged vessels

Chemotherapy — Use of drugs to kill or control cancer cells

Chronic pain — Persistent pain (more than 3–6 months), the cause of which may not be clear

Codeine	Weak opioid converted in the liver to morphine for analgesic effect
Cortico-steroids	Anti-inflammatory drugs prescribed for wide range of conditions
Nociceptive pain	Pain that is detected by specialized sensory nerves called nociceptors
Nociceptors	Specialised sensory nerve receptor cells that detect damage and irritants that cause pain and are located in muscles and skin, and internal organs
Neuropathic pain	Pain arising from damage to peripheral or central nerves or from malfunctioning of nerves
Non-opioid analgesia	Simple analgesics, often possessing anti-pyrexial or anti-inflammatory properties
Non-steroidal analgesia	Group of drugs with anti-inflammatory properties used to treat inflammation, pain or fever
Numerical rating scale	A 10 cm line divided into 1 cm notches to which patients assign a numerical value for their pain
Opioid analgesia	Synthetic drugs that bind to opioid receptors in the body to provide analgesic effect; include morphine, diamorphine, fentanyl, oxycodone
Pain	A subjective experience; what the patient says it is, existing when patient says it does
Pain threshold	Level at which individual patients feel pain
Prostaglandin	Hormone like lipid substance released at sites of tissue damage causing inflammation, pain and fever as part of the healing process
Radiotherapy	Controlled use of high energy X-rays to treat a variety of cancers
Rescue dose	Analgesic dose to be given for breakthrough pain, in addition to regular doses
Somatic pain	Nociceptive pain arising in skin and muscles
Substance P	Neurotransmitter associated with sensation of pain
Titration	Process of establishing the correct medication dose to ensure optimal pain management with minimal side effects, starting with low doses and increased until pain control is achieved

Verbal rating score	Pain assessment tool to enable patients to rate pain in association with a list of words that describe pain in terms of increasing intensity
Visceral pain	Nociceptive pain arising in the body organs or cavities
Visual analogue scale	**A** 10 cm line with descriptors of opposite pain intensity at either end; patients identify where on the line their pain exists (position reflects intensity of pain experience)
Weak opioids	Opioid-based drug that has a ceiling level, dosage maximum, includes codeine, dihydrocodeine, tramadol
WHO analgesic ladder	Advisory guidelines for prescribing and increasing analgesia appropriately

Patient scenario

Ayana Delacruz is an 80-year-old widow, who moved into residential care a year ago because she was finding it increasingly difficult to cope on her own at home. Shortly after moving into the care home, Ayana was diagnosed with lung cancer and received two weeks palliative radiotherapy which reduced her symptoms.

About two months ago, Ayana saw the GP and told her that she was experiencing a horrid pain around the bottom of her right lung. The pain was difficult to pinpoint but was very sore and uncomfortable, scoring 7–8 on the NRS. The GP diagnosed visceral pain arising from the effects of the tumour on the lung tissue and prescribed two co-codamol tablets, 6 hourly. These worked very well and Ayana's pain improved, scoring a 2 on the NRS at worst. Ayana became constipated as a result of taking the co-codamol and the GP prescribed two co-danthramer capsules nocté with good effect.

Two weeks ago Ayana experienced the severe pain again, her sleep was interrupted and her quality of life greatly reduced. Ayana stated that the pain was 7–8 again now on the NRS. The home manager asked the GP to come and review Ayana. The GP felt that the pain was still related to the lung tumour and changed Ayana's medications.

Activity 7.3

What changes do you think the GP made?

The GP increased Ayana's analgesia to 30mg of MST BD, with 10mg of oromorph for breakthrough pain. the GP also advised the staff to increase the codanthramer if Ayana becomes constipated again

Ayana's pain settled well again and she uses very little breakthrough analgesia, she is able to have her bowels open daily without needing an increase in the co-danthramer.

This week Ayana has reported quite as different pain to her carers. The pain is a deep ache and is under her right breast. One rib is particularly tender to touch. The home manager has requested another visit from the GP.

Activity 7.4

What do you think is causing Ayana's pain and what treatment do you think the GP implemented?

The GP diagnosed bone metastases in Ayana's rib. She liaised with the hospital for a one-off dose of radiotherapy and prescribed ibuprofen 400 mg 6 hourly. The GP asked the carers to observe Ayana for signs of side effects.

Gastric – abdominal pain, nausea, diarrhoea, constipation and heartburn

General – rash, ringing in the ears, headache, dizziness, drowsiness

References

Abbey, J., Piller, N., De Bellis, A., Esterman, A., Parker, D., Giles, L. and Lowcay, B. (2004) The Abbey pain scale: a 1 minute numerical indicator for people with end stage dementia. *International Journal of Palliative Nursing*. 10(1):6–13.

Bruckenthal, P. (2010) Integrating nonpharmacological and alternative strategies into a comprehensive management approach for older adults with pain. *Pain Management Nursing*. 11 (2): S23–S31.

Chapman, S. (2012) Cancer pain part 2: assessment and management. *Nursing Standard*. 26(48): 44–49.

Chatterjee, J. (2012) Improving pain assessment for patients with cognitive impairment: development of a pain assessment toolkit. *International Journal of Palliative Nursing*. 18(12): 581–590.

Dean, M.M. (2008) End of life care for COPD patients *Primary care Respiratory Journal*. 17(1): 46–50.

Estfan, B., Mahmoud, F., Shaheen, P., Davis, M.P., Lasheen, W., Rivera, N., LeGrand, S.B., Lagman, R.L., Walsh, D. and Rybicki, L. (2007) Respiratory function during parenteral opioid titration. *Palliative Medicine*. 21: 81–86.

Hall, S. (2010) Adjuvant analgesics in pain management, *Nurse Prescribing*. 8(3): 122–128.

Harlos, M. and MacDonald, L. (2005) Managing pain in palliative patients In: MacDonald, N., Oneschuk, D., Hagen, N., Doyle, D. (eds). *Palliative Medicine: A Case Based Manual* 2nd edn. Oxford: Oxford University, pp. 16–38.

Hart, J. (2008) Complementary therapies for chronic pain management. *Alternative and complementary therapies*. 14 (2): 64–68.

International Association for the Study of Pain (2012) *IASP Taxonomy* Available at http://www.iasp-pain.org/Content/NavigationMenu/GeneralResourceLinks/PainDefinitions/default.htm [accessed 17 February 2014].

International Association for the Study of Pain (1997). *Respiratory Effects of Opioids* Available at http://www.iasp-pain.org/AM/Template.cfm?Section=Technical_Corner&Template=/CM/ContentDisplay.cfm&ContentID=2196 [accessed 17 February 2014].

Lalkhen, A.B., Bedford, J.P. and Dwyer, A.D. (2012) Pain associated with multiple sclerosis: epidemiology, classification and management. *British Journal of Neuroscience*. 8(5): 267–274.

McAuliffe, L., Nay, R., O'Donnell, M. and Fetherstonhaugh, D. (2008) Pain assessment in older people with dementia: literature review. *Journal of Advanced Nursing* 65(1): 2–10.

McCaffery, M. (1968). *Nursing Practice Theories Related to Cognition, Bodily Pain, and Man-Environment Interactions*. Los Angeles: University of California at Los Angeles Students' Store.

National Institute for Health and Clinical Excellence (NICE) (2012) *Opioids in Palliative Care: Safe and Effective Prescribing of Strong Opioids for Pain in Palliative Care of Adults*. Manchester: NICE.

National Stroke Association (2012) *Pain* Available at http://www.stroke.org/site/PageServer?pagename=pain [accessed 17 February 2014].

Oliver, D., Campbell, C. and Wright, A. (2007) Palliative care of patients with motor neurone disease. *Progress in Palliative Care* 15(6): 285–93

Pattison, K.T.S. (2008) Opioids and the control of respiration. *British Journal of Anaesthesia*. 100(6): 747–58.

Russon, L. and Mooney, A. (2010) Palliative and end of life care in advanced renal failure. *Clinical Medicine* 10(3): 279–281.

Salt, S. (2003) Tripwires in palliative care In: Thomas, K. (ed). *Caring for the Dying at Home: Companions on the Journey*. Oxford: Radcliffe.

South West London Cardiac Network (2009) *Symptom Control Guidelines and Key Information in End-Stage Heart Failure*. London: South West London Cardiac Network.

Vargas-Schaffer, G. (2010) WHO analgesic ladder still valid? *Canadian Family Physician*. 56(60): 514–517.

Wheeldon, A. (2009) Pain and pain management In: Nair, M. and Peate, I. (Eds). *Fundamentals of applied pathophysiology an essential guide for nursing student*. Oxford. Wiley-Blackwell.

Williamson, A. and Hoggart, B. (2005) Pain: a review of three commonly used pain rating scales. *Issues in Clinical Nursing*. 14: 798–804.

World Health Organisation (2014) *Definitions of Palliative Care* Available at http://www.who.int/cancer/palliative/definition/en/ [accessed 17 February 2014].

8

Management and nursing care of gastro-intestinal symptoms

Introduction

Although each chronic illness will present its own specific symptoms there are some symptoms that are common to many life-limiting illnesses. Gastro-intestinal symptoms are some of the most common symptoms experienced by patients receiving palliative care, regardless of diagnosis (de Lima, 2007). Patients with different chronic diseases present with similar palliative care needs towards the end of their lives, many of which can be met by practitioners providing generic palliative care (Gadoud and Johnson, 2011). This chapter will focus on the nursing care and medical management of common gastro-intestinal symptoms.

Learning outcomes

By the end of this chapter you will be able to

- discuss the assessment of common gastro-intestinal symptoms;
- understand the principles of symptom control;
- discuss the nurse's role in symptom management.

Fundamentals of Palliative Care for Student Nurses, First Edition. Megan Rosser and Helen C. Walsh.

Companion website: www.wiley.com/go/rosser_walsh/fundamentals_of_palliative_care

Nausea and vomiting

Although generally coupled together nausea and vomiting are two separate symptoms and need to be treated as such. Studies often fail to distinguish between the two; therefore, it is difficult to accurately report the incidence of either, however nausea and or vomiting is acknowledged as one/two of the most frequent physical symptoms in palliative care (Stiel *et al.*, 2011). It has been suggested that for patients with a diagnosis of cancer the incidence of vomiting is 30% whilst the experience of nausea is 60% (Shah and Shah, 2010). The prevalence of nausea has been identified in end stage renal failure as 30% (Russon and Mooney, 2010) with the incidence of nausea ranging from 17–48% in end stage heart failure (Solano *et al.*, 2006).

What is nausea and vomiting?

Nausea An unpleasant sensation of the need to vomit, often accompanied by autonomic symptoms – pallor, sweat, salivation, tachycardia.

Vomiting The forceful expulsion of gastric content through the mouth.

Palliative Care Guidelines Plus (2013)

Pathophysiology of nausea and vomiting

Vomiting occurs in response to messages relayed from different areas of the body by neurotransmitters to the vomiting centre. If the vomiting centre is stimulated, it in turn stimulates spinal, phrenic and vagal nerves to stimulate the vomiting response. Control of vomiting is achieved by blocking the effects of the causative neurotransmitter. The various pathways involved can be seen in Figure 8.1.

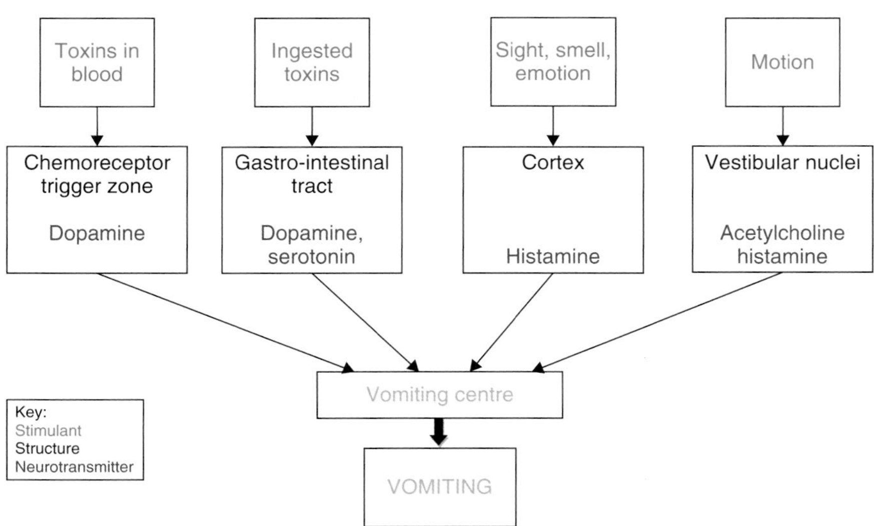

Figure 8.1 The pathophysiology of nausea and vomiting.

Table 8.1 Causes of nausea and vomiting.

Structure	Cause of vomiting
Cerebral cortex	Fear Anxiety Pain Smells Taste Increased intracranial pressure Tumour of central nervous system
CTZ	Drugs – opioids, chemotherapy Toxins – infections, radiotherapy, carcinomatosis Metabolic – uraemia, hypercalcaemia
Visceral – GI tract	Stasis – drugs, disease Squashed stomach – enlarged liver, ascites Obstruction – tumour Irritation, NSAIDs, steroids, antibiotics, chemotherapy, radiotherapy Constipation
Vestibular nuclei	Motion Labyrinthitis, ear infections Tumour on eigth cranial nerve

The key structures involved in the vomiting pathway as follows:

- the vomiting centre in the reticular formation in the brain stem;
- the chemoreceptor trigger zone (CTZ) in the area postrema;
- the cerebral cortex;
- the vestibular nuclei in the fourth ventricle.

The key neurotransmitters involved are as follows:

- Dopamine
- Histamine
- Serotonin
- Acetylcholine.

As you may realise from looking at the pathways there are numerous causes of nausea and vomiting, and the main causes are listed in Table 8.1.

Assessment

It is important to get a clear picture from the patient assessment. If the mechanism involved in the vomiting can be identified then it is easier to prescribe an appropriate anti-emetic. If the cause if unclear then a trial with a broad spectrum anti-emetic will be necessary and it may take longer to resolve the nausea or vomiting.

Activity 8.1

List the questions you would ask when assessing a patient's nausea or vomiting and compare your list to the questions in Figure 8.2.

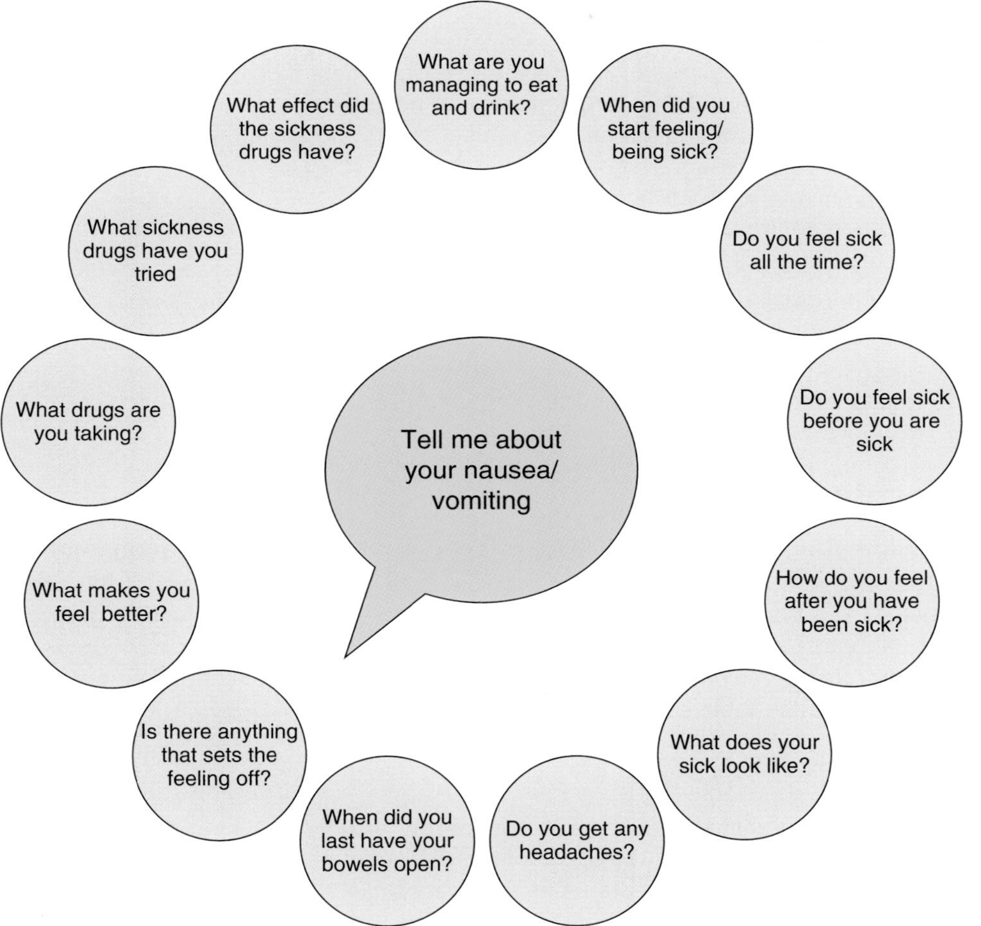

Figure 8.2 Questions to ask during an assessment of nausea and vomiting.

Important investigations that may also help determine the cause of the vomiting include

- bloods to check blood chemistry- diagnose hypercalcaemia, uraemia;
- a rectal examination to rule out constipation;
- an abdominal examination to check for enlarged liver, obstruction, ascites or constipation;
- an ultrasound to detect ascites;
- an abdominal X-ray to identify constipation.

Assessment tools such as the VAS or NRS can help the patient to communicate the severity of the nausea and vomiting from their perspective and provide baseline data for evaluating interventions.

Management of nausea and vomiting

Non-pharmacological

There are a number of non-pharmacological interventions which may help to alleviate the patient's nausea and vomiting. These include

- provision of calm, peaceful and fresh, airy environment if possible;
- explanation of examinations, diagnoses and treatments;
- emotional support and attention to patient's fears and anxieties;
- relaxation therapies;
- complementary therapies;
- appropriate preparation and presentation of food – if patient is able to eat-
    - food prepared away from patient to prevent smells stimulating nausea or vomiting response
    - offer small meals as often as patient wants
    - upright position during and after meal
- ginger is a good antiemetic- drinks, biscuits or crystallised;
- regular mouth care to keep mouth clean and fresh;
- acupuncture/acupressure- sea bands.

Pharmacological

The aim of management is to prescribe the most appropriate anti-emetic, which will relieve the nausea and vomiting by interrupting the pathway of the neurotransmitters identified in Figure 8.1. It is important to treat any reversible causes first such as infection, gastric irritation, hypercalcaemia, constipation or pain. The anti-emetics prescribed will be chosen according to the likely cause of the nausea or vomiting identified. Drugs used to control nausea and vomiting are summarised in Table 8.2 and explained in more depth now.

Cerebral cortex

If vomiting is thought to be caused by emotions then anxiolytics such as diazepam or lorazepam may help. If the patient is in pain, then pain management needs to be reviewed. If cerebral disease such as cerebral metastases or a primary brain tumour is suspected then high dose steroids will relieve some of the oedema around the tumour (s) possibly reducing the vomiting response. In order to interrupt the vomiting pathway, then anti-histamines will be prescribed; cyclizine is very effective in controlling nausea and vomiting arising from the cerebral cortex.

Chemoreceptor trigger zone (CTZ)

The CTZ is rich in dopamine receptors, and is situated on the floor of the fourth ventricle outside of the blood brain barrier; therefore, it is very susceptible to changes in blood chemistry. The CTZ may be stimulated by uraemia and hypercalcaemia or opioid drugs which the patient is using for the first time. If patients who are taking opioids for the first time experience of nausea or vomiting this is a temporary response until the CTZ gets used to the presence of the circulating opioid in the blood. This temporary experience of vomiting can be controlled by a low dose of haloperidol at night for 4–5 days. Other dopamine antagonists such as metoclopramide and haloperidol can be used if continued irritation of the CTZ is believed to be the

Table 8.2 Drugs used to control nausea and vomiting.

Structure involved	Useful drugs	Action	Side-effects
Cerebral cortex	Dexamethasone	Reduces oedema from cerebral disease	Confusion, euphoria, insomnia, fluid retention, raised blood sugars
	Cyclizine	Antihistamine – blocks histamine receptors	Drowsiness, dry mouth, confusion, urinary retention
CTZ	Haloperidol	All are dopamine antagonists	extra-pyramidal symptoms (EPS)
	Metoclopramide		EPS
	Prochlorperazine		sedating, hypotension
	Levomepromazine		sedating, hypotension
	Ondansetron, Granisetron, Tropisetron	All are serotonin antagonists	all are constipating
Gastro-intestinal tract	Metoclopramide	Increase gastric emptying	EPS
	Domperidone	Give 1/2 h before meals	EPS
	Octreotide	Reduces gastric secretions	
	Dexamethasone	Reduces oedema from tumours, reduces hepatomegaly	Confusion, euphoria, insomnia, fluid retention, raised blood sugars
	Omeprazole, Lansoprazole	Reduce gastric irritation	
Vestibular nuclei and vomiting centre	Cyclizine	Antihistamine – blocks histamine receptors	Drowsiness, dry mouth, confusion, urinary retention
	Scopolamine (patch)	Anticholinergic – blocks acetylcholine	Sedating, dry mouth, constipation, confusion, urinary retention

cause of the nausea or vomiting. The CTZ also has serotonin receptors and therefore may be stimulated by chemotherapy drugs. If this is the case, then the serotonin antagonists such as ondansetron, tropisetron or granisetron may be prescribed – these drugs are very constipating and should only be used for a few days post – chemotherapy. There is some emerging evidence that they are also useful for intractable vomiting in palliative care.

Gastro-intestinal tract

There are a number of reasons why a vomiting response may be initiated in the GI tract and each cause warrants a different treatment. If there is gastric irritation from drugs such as steroids or NSAIDs then gastric cover is required. Proton pump inhibitors such as omeprazole and lansoprazole will reduce gastric irritation. If vomiting is due to delayed gastric emptying then administering metoclopramide or domperidone (both of which are pro-kinetic drugs, i.e. they increase gastric motility) will promote gastric emptying to relieve the symptoms. Because of the action on the Mu receptors in the gut morphine can cause delayed gastric emptying in some patients. This small group of patients require regular metoclopramide for as long as they are on morphine.

Morphine also causes constipation which in turn can cause nausea and vomiting in extreme cases, so it is vital that patients on morphine receive laxative therapy as well. If squashed stomach is suspected because of an enlarged liver or ascites then steroids will reduce oedema in the liver capsule and may increase gastric capacity again. Ascites may be relieved by use of diuretics or by draining of the ascitic fluid if appropriate in accordance with the patient's wishes and prognosis.

Vestibular nuclei and vomiting centre

If the vomiting response is thought to arise in the vestibular nuclei, then regular doses of antihistamines such as cyclizine, or anti-cholinergic such as scopolamine, may relieve vomiting. In order to relieve vomiting arising from direct stimulation of the vomiting centre it is most effective to prescribe antihistamines (cyclizine) anti-cholinergic (scopolamine) or serotonin antagonists (ondansetron, tropisetron or granisetron).

If it is not possible to identify the cause then a broad spectrum anti-emetic such as levomepromazine should be prescribed. Any anti-emetic should be prescribed regularly with PRN doses as back up. It is also important that the drugs are given via the appropriate route. Oral administration is always preferable for patients but if the patient is vomiting there is absolutely no point in giving any medications orally as they will not be absorbed. Initially it may be necessary to give anti-emetics by injection or by continuous sub-cutaneous infusion via a syringe driver until vomiting is resolved.

Regular review is vital and should happen every 24 hours. If the patient's symptoms have not resolved after 24 hours it may be appropriate to add another anti-emetic with a different mechanism.

Nursing care

Activity 8.2

List the main areas of nursing care that you think are important for patients experiencing nausea/vomiting.

The main aim of nursing care for the patient who is nauseated or vomiting is to promote of comfort at all times. Some aspects of nursing care are completed in collaboration with medical staff such as continually reviewing the patient, administering antiemetics as they are prescribed and monitoring and reporting the efficacy of the drugs. From a purely nursing point of view you can assist the patient with their daily living activities as they require. In addition to maintaining fluid and diet charts and reporting any concerns, other important aspects of nursing care will include the non-pharmacological measures discussed previously. If a patient is an in-patient, encourage family members to bring in the patient's favourite foods if they are able to. If the patient is unable to tolerate fluids offer crushed ice cubes or frozen drinks. Mouth care is paramount–especially after patients have vomited and need to freshen their mouth.

Malignant bowel obstruction

Malignant bowel obstruction is a common complication for cancer patients, generally seen in patients with advanced disease when options for aggressive interventions are limited. It is most common in gynaecological cancers, especially ovarian cancer, and gastro-intestinal cancer. Other cancers than can cause an obstruction are those that metastasise to the abdomen, most commonly lung and breast cancer and malignant melanoma (Librach et al 2005). The obstruction occurs either because the gut lumen is obstructed by the tumour or gastric motility is impeded due to involvement of bowel muscle. It is likely that the specialist palliative care team will be involved in an advisory capacity to ensure optimal symptom control.

Patients in obstruction will complain of

- abdominal colic due to bowel contractions trying to overcome the obstruction;
- aching pain from the visceral pain of the tumour and abdominal distension;
- large vomits – with little nausea:
  - patient feels relieved after vomiting
  - vomit may be faecal
- constipation or reduced bowel movements;
- anorexia.

Treatment will depend on the general health of the patient and also on the anticipated prognosis. If a patient is relatively well with good prognostic factors then they may be offered a surgical bypass. Sicker patients may undergo less invasive surgical procedures such as a venting gastrostomy or stenting, which provides rapid relief for most suitable patients but is not without complications.

If the patient is too ill for surgical intervention the obstruction will be managed by a combination of drugs in a syringe driver. You may find your patients on a mixture of

- buscopan for the colic;
- diamorphine for the visceral pain;
- haloperidol and levomepromazine for the vomiting;
- octreotide to reduce gastric secretions in order to reduce the volume of the vomits.

If the obstruction is believed to be due to reduced gastric motility you may find that the specialist palliative care team has prescribed a trial of pro-kinetics such as metoclopromide to stimulate the gut. If your patient is on metoclopromide and experiences abdominal colic you must let the nurse in charge or the doctor know immediately so that the drug can be stopped. For some patients it may not be possible to relieve the vomiting completely but it is generally possible to reduce either the frequency or the volume of the vomiting, both of which are welcomed by the patient.

Constipation

Constipation is a common problem in many patients living with advanced disease, identified incidences are 53% for patients with end stage renal disease (Russon and Mooney, 2010) and 32–87% for patients with advanced cancer (Larkin *et al.*, 2008). It is also reported as frequently occurring in patients with advanced COPD and cardiac diseases (South West London Cardiac Network 2009).

What is constipation

> 'Constipation is the passage of small, hard faeces infrequently and with difficulty' Larkin *et al.* (2008: p. 798)

Activity 8.3

List the causes of constipation.

Causes of constipation

There are numerous causes of constipation, many of which are common to the advanced stages of any chronic disease. They include:

- immobility
- weakness
- fatigue
- poor diet and fluid intake
- anorexia
- environment – lacking in privacy and dignity
- drugs – morphine, diuretics, antidepressants, iron
- concurrent disease – for example, diverticulitis
- hypercalcaemia.

Assessment of constipation

Activity 8.4

List the information you would want to gather when assessing a patient's constipation.

When assessing the patient it is important to gain information about

- patient perceptions of the problem;
- environment including privacy, accessibility of facilities;
- previous bowel habits, degree of change, current situation;
- frequency and difficulty of defaecation;

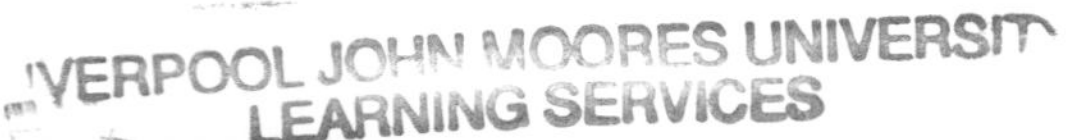

- volume and appearance of stool- blood or mucus;
- sensation of rectal fullness/satisfaction after defaecation;
- medications regime;
- aperients tried, and effect.

Larkin *et al.* (2008) and Connolly and Larkin (2012)

Tools such as the Bristol stool chart or the Norgine constipation assessment tool (Kyle, 2007) can be used to guide your assessment. In addition to your assessment the doctors will examine the patient's abdomen; they may well request an abdominal X-ray, and take blood sample to check blood chemistry to rule out conditions such as hypercalcaemia. A rectal examination is also indicated, and it is advised to adhere to the RCN (2012) guidance for this intervention.

Management of constipation

The aim of nursing care and management is to re-establish an acceptable, comfortable bowel habit and restore the patient's independence in management where possible. Medications that may be causing the patient's constipation should be changed – for example, changing oral morphine to a fentanyl patch. Oral laxatives should be used in preference to rectal interventions and the best regime is a combination of low doses of softener and stimulant.

If the patient does require rectal interventions the following may be prescribed:

Suppositories:

glycerine – softens and lubricates;
bisacodyl – stimulates.

Enemas:

arachis oil – softens (**NB** – cannot be given to people with a nut allergy as it is derived from peanut oil);
phosphate – stimulates;
sodium citrate – microlax – stimulates.

Drugs used to relieve constipation and promote regular bowel action are presented in Table 8.3.

You may see some patients whose constipation is caused by the effects of morphine prescribed methylnaltrexone (relistor) by sub-cut injection. Relistor is a peripherally-acting

mu-opioid receptor antagonist effective in tissues such as the gastrointestinal tract where it works by blocking the opioid action on GI Mu receptors (thus increasing gastric motility) without blocking central analgesic effects. The injection is generally given on alternate days but may be given each day for particularly resistant constipation (Garnock-Jones and McKeage, 2010). It is important to rotate injection sites to prevent reactions at the injection site.

Nursing care

Activity 8.5

List the nursing actions that are important when caring for someone who is constipated.

Table 8.3 Drugs used to relieve constipation.

Drug	Effect
Milpar	1–3 days Lubricates and softens stool to ease passage and stimulates peristalsis
Senna, bisacodyl	6–12 h Stimulates bowel to increase peristalsis
Docusate	1–3 days Increases penetration of water into stool- softer so easier to pass
Lactulose	1–2 days Osmotic laxative which draws fluid into the bowel thus increasing stool bulk to stimulate peristalsis Can cause wind and colic and may be unpalatable to patients because very sweet
Co-danthramer	6–12 h Combination of softener and stimulant.

Aperients such as fybogel and movicol are not recommended for palliative care patients because patients may not be able to drink the volume of fluids that have to be taken with these preparations.

Nurses are responsible for monitoring patient's bowel habits and intervening where necessary. If patients are very unwell, it is inappropriate to be advising them to increase their fibre and fluid intake or to increase their activity. For those patients who are still relatively well, these actions can be very effective in easing constipation. The administration of prescribed drugs on a regular basis will serve to promote regular bowel action. Nurses must ensure that patients are able to access toilet facilities when they need to. If patients wish to have their bowels open but are unable to get to the bathroom unaided it is vital that they are assisted, if possible, to get there to ensure maintenance of privacy and dignity. This is the case even for patients who wish to use a commode; the commode can more often than not be wheeled out. Scrupulous perineal hygiene is vital to prevent excoriation of skin or development of pressure ulcers.

If a dying patient is very restless it is advisable to check that a full bowel is not the reason for his or her distress, if it is, then suppositories or an enema may provide relief.

Cachexia

Cachexia is a significant medical problem for many patients living with chronic illnesses such as heart failure, renal disease, pulmonary disease, multiple sclerosis and cancer. Cachexia has a significant impact on patients' quality of life; it increases morbidity and mortality, exacerbates existing symptoms and is associated with a poor prognosis. Cachexia is defined as:

> 'a multifactorial syndrome characterized by severe body weight, fat and muscle loss and increased protein catabolism due to underlying disease (s)' (Muscaritoli *et al.*, 2010: p. 156)

The cause of cachexia is not fully understood but it is considered to be the result of the complex interplay between the underlying disease, disease related metabolic alterations (causing an imbalance between anabolic and catabolic processes), inflammatory responses, (primarily through the action of cytokines), and in some cases the reduced availability of nutrients (Morley *et al.*, 2006; Muscaritoli *et al.*, 2010). Cachexia is characterised by excessive involuntary weight loss, usually with disproportionate muscle wasting, decreased appetite, patients also experience significant fatigue and weakness (Morley *et al.*, 2006). Cachexia is difficult to treat, drugs such as megace, corticosteroids, cannabinoids non-steroidal anti-inflammatories and thalidomide have been used with varying success and research into effective treatment continues.

There are moves to try and provide criteria to enable staging of cachexia so that earlier intervention and possible prevention may be possible resulting in more positive outcomes if patients can be identified in the pre-cachexic state (Muscaritoli *et al.*, 2010).

Other gastrointestinal symptoms

Other gastrointestinal symptoms that may prove troublesome for patients receiving palliative care include hiccups, ascites and anorexia.

Hiccups

Hiccups result from diaphragmatic spasm and can be caused by

- gastrointestinal disorders that stimulate the vagal nerves, these disorders include reflux, gastric distension or stasis, ascites, enlarged liver, bowel obstruction;
- metabolic disorders such as uraemia;
- central nervous system tumours which affect central control of the diaphragm.

Simple traditional remedies include holding your breath, breathing into a paper bag, eating dry sugar. Medical management may be required for persistent hiccups and may include

- metoclopramide or domperidone for gastric distension or stasis;
- proton pump inhibitors for reflux;
- haloperidol if caused by uraemia;
- steroids if cause is believed to be central nervous system involvement;
- nifedepine or baclofen as muscle relaxant.

Shah and Shah (2010), Palliative care guidelines plus (2013).

Ascites

Ascites is the abnormal accumulation of fluid in the peritoneal cavity. 10% of cases develop in people living with cancer, 90% of cases arise from non-malignant diseases such as heart failure, liver failure or renal failure. The pathophysiology is not completely understood. The management of ascites falls into three categories:

- diuretics spironolactone +/− furosomide;
- paracentesis (drainage) provides temporary relief;
- perintoneo-venous shunt to drain ascitic fluid from peritoneal cavity into the superior vena cava.

Palliative care guidelines plus (2013)

Anorexia

Anorexia or loss of appetite is common in people with advanced disease, but it is different from cachexia. It can cause a lot of stress for the carers who spend time trying to make food attractive to encourage the patient to eat. Anorexia may occur because of

- pain or indigestion
- unpleasant taste in mouth
- nausea and vomiting
- metabolic causes – hypercalcaemia, uraemia
- constipation
- gastric stasis
- emotional distress
- drugs.

Many of these causes are reversible and need to be attended to in order to try and improve the patient's appetite. Other measures that will help are

- offering small, attractive meals;
- alcohol before a meal to stimulate appetite;
- referral to a dietician for advice about supplements.

Medications include steroids to increase appetite such as 4 mg dexamethasone. Any appetite stimulation from steroids is only short term. Megace, a progesterone derivative, provides a sustained increase of appetite for some patients. The recommended daily dose is 800 mg (Shah and Shah 2010; Palliative care guidelines plus, 2013).

Conclusion

Patients receiving palliative care can experience a number of different gastric symptoms, all of which can have a profound effect on the patient's quality of life. With accurate assessment of the presenting problems and multi-professional liaison about symptom control there are many pharmacological and non-pharmacological interventions that can relieve these symptoms for the patient.

Glossary

Anabolism The synthesis of molecules to build up organs and tissues, includes protein synthesis and muscle growth.

Anorexia Loss of appetite.

Antiemetic Drug used to relieve nausea and or vomiting.

Antagonist Drugs which bind to receptor cells thus blocking the action of substances such as neurotransmitters.

Anxiolytic	Drugs used primarily to relieve anxiety.
Area Postrema	Area on the floor of the fourth ventricle which receives impulses from vagal nerves and vestibular apparatus. Lies outside the blood brain barrier.
Ascites	Abnormal accumulation of fluid in the peritoneal cavity.
Blood brain barrier	A network of blood vessels with closely spaced cells that act as a filter, making it difficult for potentially toxic substances to enter the brain. Oxygen, glucose and white blood cells can pass over the barrier, red blood cells cannot.
Cachexia	Metabolic syndrome characterized by severe body weight, fat and muscle loss.
Catabolism	The breakdown of food and nutrients into smaller units, includes break down of muscle protein and fat stores.
Cerebral cortex	The surface layer of the cerebrum, composed of a thin layer of grey matter. Associated with higher level functioning including sensory perception and voluntary motor responses.
Chemoreceptor trigger zone	A group of neurons in the area postrema. Lies outside blood brain barrier and is therefore very sensitive to changes in blood chemistry. Once stimulated, it activates the vomiting centre causing vomiting.
Constipation	Passage of small, hard faeces infrequently and with difficulty.
Cytokines	Proteins that regulate various inflammatory responses.
Fourth ventricle	One of the ventricles/ cavities in the brain which produces, circulates and absorbs cerebrospinal fluid (CSF), at the same time providing a protective barrier between the CSF and the brain. Separates cerebellum from the brain stem.
Hypercalcaemia	Serum levels of calcium above 2.6mmol/l. It causes a number of symptoms including nausea and vomiting and is ultimately fatal if left untreated.
Malignant bowel obstruction	Obstruction of the bowel due to physical or mechanical obstruction.
Nausea	Unpleasant sensation of the need to vomit.
Neurotransmitter	Chemicals which allow the transmission of signals from one neuron to the next across synapses.

Prokinetic drugs	Drugs which increase gastric motility, thus speeding up gastric emptying.
Squashed stomach	Stomach unable to distend normally because of pressure from enlarged liver or ascites. Patients feel full very quickly, thus becoming anorexic and may vomit as well.
Stent	Thin metal tube placed through narrowed or blocked section of colon to relieve obstruction.
Uraemia	The presence of excess urea and other chemical waste products in the blood, caused by kidney failure in advanced disease.
Venting gastrostomy	Percutaneous endoscopic gastrostomy tube (PEG tube) inserted into the stomach through the abdominal wall to allow drainage of stomach contents in cases of malignant bowel obstruction. Drainage decompresses stomach and relieves nausea and vomiting.
Vomiting	Forceful expulsion of the gastric content through the mouth.
Vomiting centre	Located in the medulla, thereby causing emesis.
Vestibular nuclei	Collection of neurons in fourth ventricle, which are sensitive to motion and body positioning; and mediate motion sickness.

Patient scenarios

Mr Idris Llewellyn is 65 years old and has a 15 year history of ischaemic heart disease and hypertension which resulted in the development of heart failure five years ago. Mr Llewellyn lives at home with his wife and they manage well with intermittent support from the District Nurses and GP as required. Mr Llewellyn's symptoms have increased over the past six months and it is now acknowledged by all that he has end stage heart failure.

Mrs Llewellyn rang the district nurses and asked if they could visit as Mr Llewellyn was generally less well and his main problem was that he was not enjoying his food so much. Whilst the district nurse was chatting with Mr Llewellyn he remarked that he could not manage his meals as well as usual. He could only manage to eat a small amount of the food his wife prepared before he felt full. This feeling of fullness continued after meals and caused him nausea and a lot of discomfort. Mr Llewellyn also mentioned that he was sick sometimes, and when this happened the vomit contained undigested food. Mr Llewellyn felt much better after being sick. The district nurse said that she would go back to the surgery and discuss Mr Llewellyn's situation with the GP so something could be prescribed to help relieve the symptoms.

Activity 8.6

What do you think was causing Mr Llewellyn's feelings of fullness, nausea and intermittent vomiting?

What drugs do you think the district nurse might have discussed with the GP and why?

What other advice do you think she might have offered Mr and Mrs Llewellyn?

Compare your answer with the answer given below.

Squashed stomach and gastric stasis as result of intra-abdominal oedema, bowel oedema and possible hepatomegaly causing gastric congestion.

Prokinetics, to increase gastric motility and to speed up passage of food after eating. Medication to be taken half an hour before food in order to stimulate gastric motility before food is ingested.

Metoclopramide or domperidone 10-20mg TDS. GP might be cautious about prescribing domperidone as there are associations with sudden cardiac events (BNF 2013)

Advice: eat small frequent meals and snacks as opposed to trying to eat a full meal, put food on a small side plate so it looks more 'normal'

References

British National Formulary (2013) *Domperidone* Available at http://www.medicinescomplete.com/mc/bnf/current/PHP2544-domperidone.htm [accessed 18 February 2014].

Connolly, M. and Larkin, P. (2012) Managing constipation: a focus on care and treatment in the palliative setting. *British Journal of Community Nursing*. 17(2): 60–67.

De Lima, L. (2007) International Association for Hospice and Palliative Care list of essential medicines for palliative care. *Annals of Oncology*. 18(2): 395–399.

Gadoud, A.C. and Johnson, M.J. (2011) Palliative care in non-malignant disease. *Medicine* 39(11): 664–667.

Garnock-Jones, K.P., McKeage, K. (2010) Methylnaltrexone. *Drugs*. 70(7): 919–928.

Kyle, G. (2007) Norgine risk assessment tool for constipation. *Nursing Times*. 103(47): 48–49.

Larkin, P.J., Sykes, N.P., Centeno, C., Ellershaw, J.E., Elsner, F., Eugene, B., Gootjes, J.R.G., Nabal, M., Noguera, A., Ripamonti, C., Zucco, F. and Zuurmond, W.W.A. (2008) The management of constipation in palliative care: clinical practice recommendations. *Palliative Medicine* 22: 796–807.

Librach, S.L., Horvath, A.N. and Langlois, E.A. (2005) Malignant Bowel Obstruction In MacDonald, N., Oneschuk, D., Hagen, N. and Doyle D (eds) *Palliative Medicine: A Case Based Manual,* 2nd edn. Oxford: Oxford University pp. 213–227.

Morley, J.E., Thomas, D.R. and Wilson, M.M.G. (2006) Cachexia: pathophysiology and clinical relevance. *American Journal of Clinical Nutrition*. 83(4): 735–743.

Muscaritoli, M., Anker, S.D., Argiles, J., Aversa, Z., Bauer, J.M., Biolo, G., Boirie, Y., Bosaeus, I., Cederholm, T., Costelli, P., Fearon, K.C., Laviano, A., Maggio, M., Rossie-Fanelli, F., Schneider, S.M., Schols, A. and Sieber, C.C. (2010) Consensus definition of sarcopenia, cachexia and pre-cachexia: joint document elaborated by special interest groups (SIG) "cachexia-anorexia in chronic wasting diseases" and "nutrition in geriatrics". *Clinical Nutrition*. 29: 154–159.

Palliative Care Guidelines Plus (2013) Available at http://book.pallcare.info/ [accessed 18 February 2014].

Royal College of Nursing (2012) *Management of lower bowel dysfunction, including DRE and DRF. RCN guidance for nurses* Available at http://www.rcn.org.uk/__data/assets/pdf_file/0007/157363/003226.pdf [accessed 18 February 2014].

Russon, L. and Mooney, A. (2010) Palliative and end of life care in advanced renal failure. *Clinical Medicine.* 10(3): 279–81.

Shah, V. and Shah, S. (2010) Management of gastrointestinal symptoms in palliative care. *InnovAiT.* 3(7): 402–407.

Solano, J.P., Gomes, B. and Higginson, I.J. (2006) A comparison of symptom prevalence in far advanced cancer AIDS, heart disease, chronic obstructive pulmonary disease and renal disease. *Journal of Pain and Symptom Management.* 31(1): 58–69.

South West London Cardiac Network (2009) *Symptom Control Guidelines and Key Information in End-Stage Heart Failure*. London: South West London Cardiac Network.

Stiel, S., Hollberg, C., Pestinger, M., Ostgathe, C., Nauck, F., Lindena, G., Elsner, F. and Radbruch, L. (2011) Subjective definitions of problems and symptoms in palliative care. *Palliative care: research and treatment.* 5: 1–7.

9

Management and nursing care of breathlessness and fatigue

Introduction

Breathlessness and fatigue are two of the most prevalent symptoms experienced by patients living with chronic disease. Both symptoms impact at the physical, emotional and spiritual levels and if left untreated can severely compromise patients' quality of life, preventing them from getting on with their lives for the time that is left. Persistent or worsening breathlessness and fatigue gives rise to a sense of helplessness and frustration. Treatment of either symptom may involve identification and correction of the cause or purely the palliation of the presenting symptom. This chapter considers causes and management of both these troublesome symptoms.

Learning outcomes

By the end of this chapter you will be able to

- identify the common causes of breathlessness and fatigue;
- discuss the assessment of breathlessness and fatigue;
- discuss medical management of breathlessness and fatigue;
- discuss the appropriate nursing care for patients living with either symptom.

Fundamentals of Palliative Care for Student Nurses, First Edition. Megan Rosser and Helen C. Walsh.

Companion website: www.wiley.com/go/rosser_walsh/fundamentals_of_palliative_care

Breathlessness

Breathlessness, otherwise known as dyspnoea, is a common and persistent symptom for many people living with advanced chronic disease. Breathlessness increases as diseases progress and end of life approaches and can be very frightening for patients, families and healthcare professionals. Patients with non-cancer diagnoses have been found to experience significantly higher levels of breathlessness towards the end of their disease than patients with cancer diagnosis (Currow *et al.*, 2010). The pattern of breathlessness also changes with diagnosis: patients with cardiopulmonary illnesses experience severe breathlessness for longer periods than patients with cancer and the experience of breathlessness rises rapidly in cancer patients in the last few days of life (Breaden, 2011). The incidence of breathlessness for different patient groups can be seen in Fact Box 9.1.

Fact Box 9.1

Incidence of breathlessness for different patient groups- % of patients experiencing breathlessness

COPD	98%
Heart failure	88%
MND	85%
Cancer	Up to 70%

Olivier *et al.* (2007), Dean (2008), Gysels and Higginson (2011)

What is breathlessness?

Breathlessness has been described by the American Thoracic Society (ATS) (1999) as a 'subjective experience of breathing discomfort', and, therefore, it is vital that the assessment of breathlessness focuses on the patient's perspective as opposed to the professional's interpretation. The ATS (1999) also states that the experience of breathlessness includes physical, psychological, emotional and environmental factors, so holistic assessment is paramount.

Pathophysiology of breathlessness

The physiology of normal breathing is covered in another book in this series (Wheeldon, 2009). The pathophysiology of breathlessness is poorly understood but thought to result from one of the three abnormalities that occur within the process of respiration (Indelicato, 2006).

- an increase in the respiratory effort required – occurs in obstructive or restrictive lung disease;
- an increase in the proportion of respiratory muscle needed to maintain normal respiration, as the result of muscular weakness – occurs in neurological disease and advanced disease;
- increased respiratory requirements due to changes in blood chemistry – occurs with anaemia, uraemia.

Patients may experience all three at the same time in differing degrees.

Activity 9.1

List all the reasons you can think of because of which a patient with advanced disease might be breathless.

Causes of breathlessness

There are a number of causes of breathlessness, most relating to cardiopulmonary pathology and some systemic causes. Causes include the following:

- progressive airflow obstruction;
- collapse of small airways;
- reduced lung volume – pulmonary oedema, effusions, ascites;
- muscle weakness;
- changes in the blood chemistry altering response of the respiratory receptors, anaemia, uraemia.

Assessment of breathlessness

Because of the subjective nature of breathlessness it is vital that the patient's perspective forms the basis of the assessment rather than professional judgement. The experience of breathlessness tends to vary between patients with different diagnoses but like a comprehensive pain assessment there are key questions that should be asked.

Activity 9.2

List the questions you would ask when assessing a breathless patient and compare them to those in Figure 9.1.

Assessment tools

There are not many assessment tools for breathlessness but visual analogue scales and numerical rating scales have been found to be useful. Specialist palliative care teams may use more complex assessment tools such as the modified Borg scale, the chronic respiratory questionnaire, dyspnoea subscale or the Japanese Cancer Dyspnoea Scale (Dorman *et al.*, 2007).

Pharmacological Management of breathlessness

Any treatable exacerbating condition should be addressed as appropriate (depending on the patient's prognosis), for example anaemia or chest infection. Patients should continue with their prescribed drugs if still beneficial. These may include bronchodilators, ACE inhibitors, and diuretics.

When did this episode start?*
How does your breathlessness affect your life?
When do you feel breathless?
What drugs have you tried?
What effect did they have?
Tell me about your breathlessness
How would you describe your breathlessness?
What makes it worse?
Can you rate your breathlessness?
(best and worst)
What makes it better?
Do you have any other symptoms
(cough)

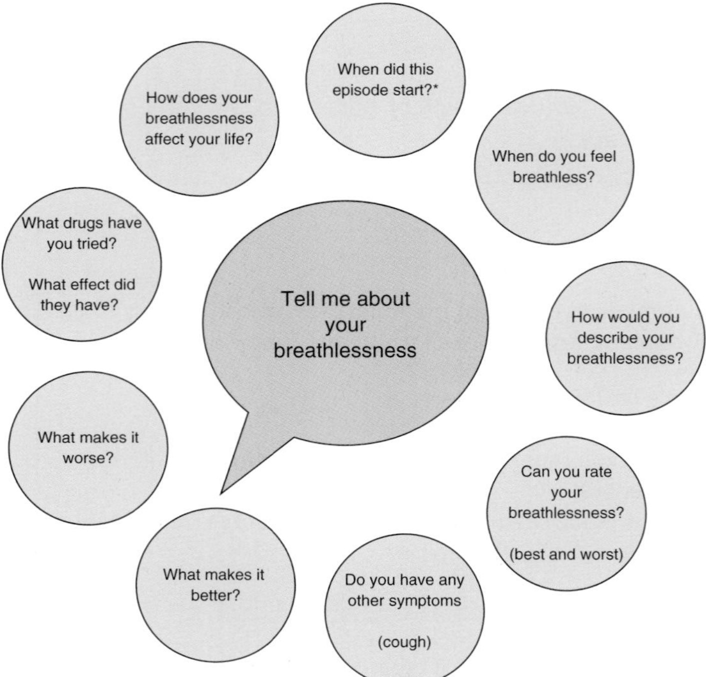

*Patients with long standing cardiac or respiratory disease may find this hard to answer because the onset of breathlessness is insidious and may have been experienced for years

Figure 9.1 Questions to be asked during assessment of breathlessness.

Opioids are the gold standard for managing breathlessness (Breaden, 2011). When titrated to the level of breathlessness that the patient is experiencing opioids will not shorten patients' lives and may in fact prolong their life because of relief of symptoms. Morphine should be given orally or sub-cutaneously, nebulised morphine has been used in some practices but this has not been proved to be clinically beneficial. Sustained release morphine such as MST is the drug of choice. It is important to observe patients for side effects and treat accordingly.

Oxygen is only useful for patients whose breathlessness is related to hypoxia and patients with sats of less than 92% when breathing room air may benefit (NICE, 2010). Patients may undergo a trial of 3–4 days to see if they benefit, if there is no improvement, then oxygen therapy should be stopped (Breaden, 2011). If patients have been prescribed oxygen this should be delivered via nasal cannulae where possible, cannulae are better tolerated by most patients and do not create the same barrier as an oxygen mask. Stringent mouth care will be required, breathless patients are likely to mouth breathe and thus the mucous membranes will dry out rapidly. If oxygen is given via a mask it also dries out the mucous membrane. If oxygen is given via nasal cannulae the nostrils must be kept clean, hydrated and comfortable.

Anxiolytics such as diazepam or lorazepam may be given to help to relieve the anxiety associated with feelings of breathlessness. Steroids are useful if breathlessness is related to major airway obstruction such as superior vena cava. Bronchodilators are likely to have already been prescribed for cardio-pulmonary patients but may be introduced to overcome airflow obstruction in patients with other diseases such as cancer.

Nursing management

Activity 9.3

List the nursing interventions that can help ease a patient's breathlessness.

In addition to medical efforts to relieve patients' breathlessness, there are a number of effective nursing and non-pharmacological interventions. In the late 1990s, a group of nurses from the Royal Marsden Hospital undertook a number of studies on the impact of specific nursing interventions on the experience of breathlessness of cancer patients.

Interventions included the following:

- helping patients address the emotional impact of their disease, the experience of breathlessness and associated deterioration;
- introducing behavioural and cognitive strategies to help them cope with their breathlessness;
- activity pacing;
- goal planning;
- breathing retraining;
- relaxation;
- panic management strategies;
- helping family members to develop supportive skills such as relaxation techniques, breathing techniques;
- helping patients and families recognise medical problems which would require attention – such as chest infections, pleural effusions.

These interventions were found to benefit patients and can be used in conjunction with medical interventions (Krishnasamy *et al.*, 2001). These nursing interventions have now been extended to patients with diagnoses other than cancer.

Positioning of the breathless patient is important. Breathless patients prefer to sit upright in order to expand their lung capacity and reduce the effort of breathing. Some patients may prefer to stay sitting in a comfortable chair rather than being nursed in bed where they may fear slipping down into a position that makes breathing more difficult. If that is the case then the most comfortable chair should be sought, pressure saving devices used and regular pressure area care provided. Patients are at great risk of developing pressure ulcers because they are generally unwell and they are sitting still for long periods and may be hypoxic and/or malnourished.

If the patient needs to move, it is best to use a wheelchair in order to preserve their energy levels. Use of a commode may be easier for the patient than walking to the toilet. Once the patient is on the commode it is preferable, if at all possible, to wheel the patient out to the toilet for privacy.

If possible the patient should be nursed in a well ventilated room; this can lessen the sensation of breathlessness. Use of a fan has been found to be helpful. In addition to physical management, psychological support is also very important and is discussed in more detail in Chapter 10.

Fatigue

Fatigue is a symptom frequently experienced by patients with progressive life-threatening illnesses and has a major impact on the quality of life. The symptom of fatigue varies across the diagnostic groups, both in terms of incidence and experience. The incidence of fatigue is shown in Fact Box 9.2:

Fact Box 9.2

Incidence of fatigue in patients – % of patients experiencing fatigue according to diagnostic group:

COPD	96%
MS	80%
End stage heart failure	75–80%
CKD	71%
Cancer	70%+

Giovannoni (2006), Jansenn *et al.* (2008), Dean (2008), Russon and Mooney (2010), Spichiger *et al.* (2012)

What is fatigue?

Activity 9.4

Have a go at describing the sensation of fatigue.

There is no single definition of fatigue and it is acknowledged that fatigue in illness is different from fatigue experienced by healthy people. Fatigue associated with illness cannot be relieved by reduced activity or increased rest and sleep. It can be unremitting with a significant impact on patients' quality of life (Ream, 2007). Fatigue may be physical or cognitive and, therefore, impinges on most aspects of life and can be extremely disabling.

A definition is offered by Radbruch *et al.* (2008: p. 15) as

> 'a subjective feeling of tiredness, weakness or lack of energy'

Causes

Activity 9.5

List factors that you think might cause fatigue.

The physiological responses that cause fatigue in advanced disease are not fully understood, and it is thought to relate either to inflammatory responses or imbalances in the function of the nervous system (Hawthorn, 2010). Factors that compound levels of fatigue include

- treatment
- disease progression
- anaemia
- weight loss
- malnutrition and dehydration
- organ failure
- altered blood chemistry
- inactivity
- drug side effects
- comorbidity

Assessment

There is wide spread agreement that fatigue is not treated as a significant symptom by many practitioners because it is presumed to be inevitable in advanced diseases. For this reason healthcare professionals do not focus on it and patients do not think of reporting it; hence, fatigue is poorly assessed and managed (Ream, 2007; Radbruch *et al*, 2008; Hawthorn, 2010).

Fatigue is multi-dimensional, so needs to be assessed holistically, paying sufficient attention to all aspects of the experience. Asking the patient to tell you about their tiredness and the impact it has on their lives gives them permission to talk about their experience. It enables you as a nurse to listen and pick out the key issues for the patient. Because of the subjective nature, patient self reporting is again the most appropriate assessment method.

Activity 9.6

List the questions you would ask the patient.

It is helpful to ask the patient a number of questions:

- how would they describe their fatigue?
- what they can and cannot do – physically, cognitively, emotionally?
- is there any pattern to their fatigue?
- what makes it better/worse?
- how does it make them feel?

There are formal tools which can be used to help in the assessment – a simple VAS or NRS enables the patient to communicate the severity of their experience. Focussed tools such as the brief fatigue inventory and the fatigue assessment questionnaire may be used (Hawthorn, 2010).

Management of fatigue

Pharmacological management

It is important that reversible causes such as anaemia, infection and dehydration are treated; if that is appropriate according to the patient's prognosis. Drugs that may be exacerbating the fatigue should be stopped if possible, morphine doses and the use of drugs such as benzodiazepines may need reviewing. Attention must be paid to other symptoms such as sleeplessness to enable these to be managed appropriately.

Medical interventions for fatigue are of limited benefit, regimes may differ according to the patient's underlying disease. Currently there is no agreed strategy for optimal management; the more common drug treatment is short term use of steroids. The use of stimulants such as methylphenidate and modafinil lacks a strong evidence base and is, therefore, controversial (Radbruch *et al.*, 2008).

Non-pharmacological management

More progress has been made in the non-pharmacological management of patients' fatigue and effective interventions include

- provision of information about how to manage fatigue;
- maintaining a diary to establish patterns of fatigue;
- carefully calibrated exercise regimes to conserve and restore energy levels;
- counselling to identify coping strategies;
- relaxation;
- pacing of activities;
- complementary therapies;
- acupuncture and acupressure.

Ream (2007), Radbruch *et al* (2008), Jones and Elbert-Avila (2011)

Nursing care

Activity 9.7

List the nursing interventions you think would be appropriate for fatigued patients.

The role of the nurse when supporting fatigued patients is paramount; you can assist them with their activities of daily living as required. It is important not to take over but to work with the patient to help them maintain independence where possible, assisting with activities that they are unable to complete themselves.

Nursing care will include

- assisting with personal hygiene needs;
- manual handling assessment;

- maintaining patient mobility through the use of mobility aids;
- monitoring patient's elimination – they may become constipated as a result of fatigue;
- helping with eating and drinking if the patients are too tired to feed themselves – maintaining food and fluid charts as appropriate;
- promoting a good night's sleep;
- providing emotional support as required;
- preventing complications of immobility, use of pressure saving devices, regular pressure area care, monitoring bowel movements.

Conclusion

Breathlessness and fatigue are both debilitating symptoms experienced by patients during their disease trajectories, and the symptoms are increasing for many as they approach end stage. Both symptoms have considerable subjective components and impact significantly on the patients' quality of life. Pharmacological interventions are of limited benefit to patients and nursing support and non-pharmacological interventions have been proven to provide relief for many patients.

Glossary

ACE inhibitors	Angiotensin-converting enzyme inhibitors – used to treat high blood pressure and heart failure.
Activity pacing	Helping patients to plan their days, prioritising tasks, spreading out demanding activities and planning rest periods so they can rest before they become tired.
Anaemia	Reduction in red blood cells and or haemoglobin, reducing the blood's ability to transport oxygen around the body.
Anxiolytic	Drugs used primarily to relieve anxiety.
Ascites	Abnormal accumulation of fluid in the peritoneal cavity.
Breathing retraining	Helping the patient to learn a new efficient breathing pattern to maximise lung capacity, reduce anxiety and effort and facilitate a reduction in respiratory rate.
Breathlessness	Subjective experience of breathing discomfort.
Bronchodilators	Medications which make breathing easier by relaxing the muscles in the lungs and widening the airways.
Cognitive strategies	Different ways of thinking about/ coping with things such as breathlessness and fatigue.

Comorbidity	Two or more co-existing diseases.
Dyspnoea	The distressing awareness of the process of breathing.
Fatigue	A subjective feeling of tiredness, weakness or lack of energy.
Hypoxic	Low levels of oxygen circulating in the blood.
Opioids	Synthetic drugs that bind to opioid receptors in the body, including the cardiovascular system, so may be used to relieve sensation of breathlessness.
Panic management strategies	Helping patients to learn how to manage sensations of panic, includes relaxation, breathing and thinking about things differently.
Pleural effusion	Build up of fluid in the potential space between the pleura which line the thoracic cavity.
Pressure ulcers	Breakdown of skin and underlying tissue due to interrupted blood supply as the result of prolonged pressure. The affected skin becomes starved of oxygen and nutrients and begins to break down, leading to an ulcer forming.
Pulmonary oedema	Accumulation of fluid in the lungs, often due to heart failure or renal failure.
Respiratory effort	The amount of effort used to breathe, normal breathing is effortless.
Uraemia	The presence of excess urea and other chemical waste products in the blood, caused by kidney failure in advanced disease.

Patient scenario

Fiona Turner is a 48-year-old married lady who has lived with relapsing, remitting, multiple sclerosis for the past 15 years. Both her children are away at University. Fiona has experienced relapses over the course of her illness, receiving support from the MS nurse and the district nurse. Fiona recovers well and has had very little time off from her job as a manager in the local council's human resources department.

Recently Fiona has noticed that she has been becoming increasingly tired, falling asleep on the sofa when she gets in from work, instead of her normal routine of taking the dog out for a walk. Fiona has not felt like going to her regular yoga class for weeks. In the past two weeks she has felt overwhelmingly fatigued, this feeling of fatigue is not relieved by rest or sleep. Fiona is contemplating taking some time off work, she is finding it increasingly difficult to concentrate and her memory is getting worse. Fiona is also aware that some of her previous symptoms are beginning to emerge; she has been experiencing some visual disturbances and feels her balance is compromised at times. Fiona is finding it increasingly difficult to keep going, she fears a relapse and has asked the district nurse to visit her to discuss her fears and to ask for advice regarding managing the fatigue.

Activity 9.8

What advice do you think the district nurse could give regarding managing Fiona's fatigue?

Compare your answers with those below.

Answer:

1. Rule out reversible causes that may be exacerbating fatigue- eg urinary tract infection, respiratory infection.
2. Advice:
   - Keeping a diary of the episodes of fatigue- enables Fiona to establish a pattern, possibly identifying any triggers that could be avoided in future.
   - Attention to sleep patterns-
     attend to any symptoms that may be interrupting sleep-pain, spasm, micturition.
     try and establish bedtime routine with regular hours of sleep, avoid stimulant drinks such as caffeine in the evening.
     encourage Fiona to continue to exercise to help her sleep.
   - Nutritional advice-
     well balanced diet, adequate hydration.
   - Attention to mood.
   - Stress avoidance/ management.
   - Relaxation-
     reathing or visualisation exercises, complementary therapies.
   - Exercise-
     encourage Fiona to continue with exercise which she is able to do, inactivity exacerbates fatigue. Encourage gentle exercise, such as walking the dog, with rests as necessary.
   - Pacing and prioritising of activities-
     maximises energy and ensures most efficient use of energy.
3. Refer to the MS nurse specialist for review in case of possible relapse.

References

American Thoracic Society (1999) Dyspnea: mechanisms, assessment and management: a consensus statement. *American Journal of Critical Care Medicine.* 159: 321–340.

Breaden, K. (2011) Recent advances in the management of breathlessness. *Indian Journal of Palliative Care.* S29–S32 - S = supplement.

Currow, D.C., Smith, J., Davidson, P.M., Newton, P.J., Agar, M.R. and Abernethy, A.P. (2010) Do the trajectories of dyspnea differ in prevalence and intensity by diagnosis at the end of life? A consecutive cohort study. *Journal of Pain and Symptom Management.* 39(4): 680–690.

Dean, M.M. (2008) End of life care for COPD patients. *Primary Care Respiratory Journal.* 17(1): 46–50.

Dorman, S., Byrne, A. and Edwards, A. (2007) Which measurement tools should we use to ensure breathlessness in palliative care? A systematic review. *Palliative Medicine.* 21: 177–191.

Giovannoni, G. (2006) Multiple sclerosis related fatigue. *Journal of Neurology, Neurosurgery and Psychiatry.* 77(1): 2–3.

Gysels, M.H. and Higginson, I.J. (2011) The lived experience of breathlessness and its implications for care: a qualitative comparison in cancer COPD heart failure and MND. *Biomed central palliative care.* Available at http://www.biomedcentral.com/content/pdf/1472-684X-10-15.pdf [accessed 19 February 2014].

Hawthorn, M. (2010) Fatigue in patients with advanced cancer. *International Journal of Palliative Nursing* 16(11): 536–541.

Indelicato, R.A. (2006) The advanced practice nurse's role in palliative care and the management of dyspnea. *Topics in Advanced Practice Nursing ejournal* 6(4) Available at http://www.medscape.com/viewarticles/551364_print [accessed 19 February 2014].

Jansenn, D.J.A., Spruit, M.A., Woulters E.F.M. and Schols J.M.G.A. (2008) Daily symptom burden in end stage chronic organ failure: a systematic review. *Palliative Medicine* 22: 938–948.

Jones, C.A. and Elbert-Avila, K. (2011) Palliative care in advanced cancer in older adults: management of pain, fatigue, and gastrointestinal symptoms. *Clinical Geriatrics.* 19 (11): 23–9.

Krishnasamy, M., Corner, J., Bredin, M., Plant, H. and Bailey, C. (2001) Cancer nursing practice development: understanding breathlessness. *Journal of Clinical Nursing.* 10: 103–108.

National Institute for Health and Clinical Excellence (NICE) (2010) *Chronic obstructive pulmonary disease - Management of chronic obstructive pulmonary disease in adults in primary and secondary care.* London: NICE.

Olivier, D., Campbell, C. and Wright, A. (2007) Palliative care of patients with motor neurone disease. *Progress in Palliative Care.* 15(6): 285–93.

Radbruch, L., Strasser, F., Elsner, F., Gonclaves, J.F., Loge, J., Kassa, S., Nauck, F. and Stone, P. (2008) Fatigue in palliative care: an EAPC approach. *Palliative Medicine.* 22: 13–32.

Ream, E. (2007) Fatigue in patients receiving palliative care. *Nursing Standard.* 21 (28): 49–56.

Russon, L. and Mooney, A. (2010) Palliative and end of life care in advanced renal failure. *Clinical Medicine* 10(3): 279–81.

Spichiger, E., Muller-Frohlich, C., Denhaerynck, K., Stoll, H., Hantikainen, V., Dodd, M. (2012) Prevalence and contributors to fatigue in individuals hospitalised with advanced cancer: a prospective, observational study. *International Journal of Nursing Studies.* 49: 1146–1154.

Wheeldon, A. (2009) The respiratory system and associated disorders In Nair, M. and Peate I. (eds) *Fundamentals of Applied Pathophysiology An Essential Guide for Nursing Student.* Oxford: Wiley-Blackwell.

10

Management and nursing care of psychological symptoms

Introduction

The NMC (2010) expects newly qualified nurses to be competent to make an holistic, person-centred assessment of a patient, which includes not only their physical condition, but also their emotional, psychological, social and cultural needs. Whilst the assessment and management of pain and other distressing physical symptoms have traditionally been the focus of the end of life care (Agrawal and Danis, 2002), psychological symptoms such as depression and anxiety consistently rank in the top five symptoms experienced by patients receiving palliative care. Often far more challenging and complex, psychological symptoms can sometimes receive less attention, while health care professionals (HCPs) concentrate on the physical aspects of palliation (Amoah, 2011). This chapter seeks to identify the nurse's role in assessing, caring for and supporting patients experiencing psychological symptoms.

Fundamentals of Palliative Care for Student Nurses, First Edition. Megan Rosser and Helen C. Walsh.

Companion website: www.wiley.com/go/rosser_walsh/fundamentals_of_palliative_care

Learning outcomes

By the end of this chapter you should be able to

- understand the importance of recognising psychological symptoms;
- consider how physical and psychological symptoms can impact on each other;
- identify common psychological symptoms;
- discuss the nurse's role in responding to psychological symptoms.

Activity 10.1

Think of a patient you have looked after who has been receiving palliative care. Try and put yourself in his/her position. What concerns, worries or anxieties do you think he/she may have had or that you might have in that position?

Your list might have contained some of the questions listed in Box 10.1.

Box 10.1 Questions someone receiving palliative care may ask

What's going to happen to me? Will it hurt? Why me? Why now?
What treatment can I have? Will it work? Will there be side effects?
What will people think about me?
Who should I tell? How will I tell them? How can anyone still love me?
Will I die? How will I die? When will I die? Where will I die?
Will my family cope? Will they cope with my illness? And afterwards?
What about money? Will the money go far enough? Who is going to pay for my funeral? How will my family manage financially?
How am I going to cope with all these losses? Loss of control; loss of my role; my health; home; loss of dignity?

Basically these can be summed up as concerns about

- the illness;
- possible treatment, effectiveness and side effects;
- the future;
- existential concerns.

All these concerns have an impact on the patient's psychological well being, which in turn affects their physical wellbeing. It is, therefore, important that a biopsychosocial approach to assessment and management is taken. The term 'opioid-irrelevant pain' is often used to describe pain that does not respond to analgesics, reminding us that different strategies are needed for their management (IASP, 2009). The factors affecting pain thresholds were discussed in Chapter 7, the majority of the factors were directly related to psychological issues.

Palliative care patients often have a number of physical symptoms which can contribute to psychological distress. The relationship between the number and severity of physical symptoms is often a predictor of psychological distress such as anxiety and depression (Dudgeon *et al.*, 2012). A definition of psychological distress is shown in Fact Box 10.1.

Fact Box 10.1

A definition of psychological distress

Psychological distress is a multi-factorial unpleasant emotional experience of a psychological (cognitive, behavioural, emotional, social and/or spiritual) nature that may interfere with the ability to cope with illness or its consequences. Distress extends along a continuum, ranging from sadness and fears to problems that can become disabling, such as depression, anxiety, panic, social isolation and existential and spiritual crises.

(Adapted from National Comprehensive Cancer Network (NCCN) (2010))

Good and effective palliative care involves attending to the whole patient and that involves their psychological needs. A definition for psychological care is shown in Fact Box 10.2.

Fact Box 10.2

Definition of psychological care

Psychological care is concerned with the psychological and emotional well being of the patient and their family/carers, including issues of self esteem, insight into an adaptation to the illness and its consequences, communication, social functioning and relationships.

(National Council of Hospice and Specialist Palliative Care Services (1997))

Psychological concerns

Sadness and anger

Sadness and anger can result from all the losses a patient experiences from the initial diagnosis, through treatment, relapse and deterioration to death. These losses include things such as independence, future, roles and changes to those roles. For example, the patient may still be a mother, but if she can no longer take the children to school or cook their meals then the role needs redefining. The new role may not be as satisfying. Whilst disfigurement and body changes resulting from the disease or treatments may be immediately apparent, we must not forget the subtle changes that accompany chronic disease, for example changes in skin texture, weight gain/loss, multiple medication, fatigue. These can have a dramatic effect on the patient and their psychological needs. Indeed, the weakness and sense of helplessness which goes with chronic illness, is in itself frightening (Macleod, 2007). These factors may lead to the patient feeling both sad and angry.

Activity 10.2

Spend a few moments reflecting on a patient you have nursed with advanced disease. Were they sad or angry? Did you recognise these emotions at the time? Would you care for them differently now, and if so, in what ways?

Allowing sadness and anger to be expressed can alleviate some of the distress they cause. Use of effective communication skills allows patients the opportunities to verbalise their fears, their sense of hopelessness and helplessness which may then relieve some of the psychological distress contributing to their 'total' pain.

Depression and Anxiety

A common mistake when caring for those receiving palliative care is to assume that anxiety and depression are normal, natural reactions to an incurable illness. Although psychological adjustment reactions after diagnosis or relapse often include fear, sadness and anger, these generally resolve within a few weeks with the help of the patient's own resources, family support and in some cases professional care (Barraclough, 1997). It is important, however, to recognise psychiatric disorders because if they go unrecognised and consequently untreated, they add to the patient's distress. Some of the reasons why anxiety and depression go unrecognised are shown in Box 10.2.

Box 10.2 Reasons for overlooking anxiety and depression (NHS Lothian, 2010)

- Patients are reluctant to express these concerns often because they are frightened of the stigma of mental health issues or scared of being perceived as 'weak'.
- Professionals are reluctant to inquire about them often because of lack of time, lack of skill or emotional self protection.
- Attributing somatic symptoms to the disease rather than considering underlying anxiety or depression.
- Assumption that any emotional distress is inevitable and also untreatable.
- Patients and family want to maintain the 'fighting spirit' and must not give in.
- Concerns about polypharmacy and drug interactions.

Activity 10.3

Spend a few minutes thinking about what you understand by the terms anxiety and depression.

Anxiety and depression are broad terms which cover a continuum of emotional states (Barraclough, 1997). Sometimes they occur together, but for ease of discussion they will now be explored separately.

Anxiety

Anxiety is a term used to describe both a symptom and a variety of psychiatric disorders in which, it is a dominant symptom (Stoklosa *et al.*, 2007). These disorders are shown in Box 10.3 and a definition of anxiety itself is offered in Fact Box 10.3. It is a common symptom for those facing life threatening illness, 25% of cancer patients and 50% of those with COPD and CHF experience anxiety (Stoklosa *et al.*, 2007). Unrecognised and untreated anxiety can become severe and disabling (Lloyd-Williams, 2004).

Box 10.3 Anxiety disorders

Generalised anxiety disorder Characterised by pervasive and excessive anxiety and worry about events or activities occurring for more days than not for at least six months. At least three of the following symptoms are present: restlessness, fatigue, difficulty concentrating, irritability, muscle tension and sleep disturbance.

Adjustment disorder Occurs within three months of a major stressor and causes marked distress and impairment of function.

Acute or post traumatic stress disorders Occur after a traumatic life event and is characterised by anxiety, arousal, numbness, flashbacks, intrusive thoughts and avoidance of stimuli which remind the patient of the trauma.

Fact Box 10.3

Definition of anxiety

Anxiety can be defined as a state of apprehension and fear resulting from the perception of a current or future threat to oneself (Stoklosa *et al.*, 2007).

Anxiety is a normal emotion, which may increase at diagnosis, with progression of the illness and when new symptoms appear or existing ones get worse (Lloyd-Williams, 2003). There are a number of causes of anxiety in patients receiving palliative care. For example, it is a prominent

Box 10.4 Manifestations of anxiety (Lloyd-Williams, 2003)

Classification	Symptoms
Psychological	Apprehension, worry, inability to relax, difficulty in concentrating, irritability, difficulty in falling asleep, unrefreshing sleep and nightmares
Motor tension	Muscular aches and fatigue, restlessness, trembling, jumpiness, tension headaches
Autonomic	shortness of breath, palpitations, lightheadedness, dizziness, sweating, dry mouth 'lump in throat', nausea, diarrhoea and frequency of urination
Physical symptoms include	Headaches, breathlessness, gastrointestinal symptoms and 'lump in throat'.
Behaviours	Behaviours include tearfulness, preoccupation, changes in sleep and eating patterns

component of physical symptoms such as chronic pain, breathlessness and nausea, whilst existential and psychosocial concerns relating to death, dying, loss and disability can also be contributory factors (Stoklosa *et al.*, 2007).

Along with behaviours, symptoms of anxiety can be considered under the following headings: psychological, motor tension, autonomic and physical. These are shown in Box 10.4.

Depression

Depression is the commonest mental health problem in palliative care. Whilst it is an illness characterised by prolonged low mood affecting the ability to carry out day to day activities, there is no universal definition of depression in the medically sick (Lawrie *et al.* 2004). Perhaps this is one of the reasons it often goes undiagnosed and undertreated in palliative care (Lloyd-Williams and Payne, 2003). Whilst 20–30% of palliative care patients will have depression, up to 80% of cases are untreated (Lawrie *et al.*, 2004;). Some of the reasons for this are shown in Box 10.5.

Depression is characterised by a variety of symptoms (Lloyd-Williams and Payne, 2003). These symptoms are summarised in Box 10.6.

Box 10.5 Reasons why depression is not treated.

- Seen as appropriate reaction to diagnosis/prognosis.
- Belief that all dying patients are depressed.
- It is an all important part of coming to terms with the illness and death.
- Health care professionals are unwilling to cause upsetting the patient by asking
- Antidepressant therapy is considered inappropriate.
- Patients do not want to admit to feeling depressed.

Box 10.6 Signs and symptoms of depression (NHS Lothian, 2010; Lawire *et al.*, 2004)

Physical symptoms	**AND in addition to these physical symptoms**
Reduced energy and fatigue (42%)	Low mood present for most of the time characteristically worse in the mornings (78%)
Disturbed sleep, especially early morning waking	Indecisiveness
Appetite/weight change either increase and gain or reduction and loss	Loss of interest, motivation or pleasure
Psychomotor slowing or agitation	Impaired ability to concentrate, think and make decisions
Decreased libido	Feelings of guilt, worthlessness or shame (50%)
Constipation	Pessimistic or hopeless ideas about the future (56%)
Disturbed and unrefreshing sleep	Suicidal thoughts or acts
Delusions	Social withdrawing
Hallucinations	A positive response to the question 'Do you feel depressed?'

Diagnosing depression is difficult because the physical symptoms overlap those of advanced illness. The patient complains of somatic symptoms and the cause is attributed to the physical illness, resulting in psychological distress being overlooked. The perceived severity of these physical symptoms may be disproportionate to that normally expected from the physical causes alone and they tend to have a poor response to medical treatments if underlying psychological factors are ignored (NHS Lothian, 2010). When psychological distress is acknowledged, it is important to exclude a severe adjustment reaction such as sadness or anxiety.

Box 10.7 compares the symptoms of an adjustment reaction with depression alone.

Box 10.7 Comparison between a severe adjustment reaction and depression

Adjustment reaction	**Depression alone**
Loss of interest	Loss of all emotion and pleasure in life
Decreased concentration	Social withdrawal
Tearfulness	Not distractible
Anxiety	Diurnal variation
Decreased sleep	Hopelessness/worthlessness
Tiredness	Excessive guilt
Anorexia	Intractable pain
Suicidal ideas	Requests for euthanasia
	Suicide attempts
	Delusions/hallucinations

Box 10.8 DSMIV (American Psychiatric Association 1994)

Core Symptoms	**Other symptoms**
Depressed mood	Changes in weight and appetite, and fatigue
Decreased interest or pleasure in activities	Changes in sleep patterns
Worthlessness or excessive/inappropriate guilt	Psychomotor agitation or retardation
Decreased ability to concentrate or indecisive	Loss of energy
Recurrent thoughts of death and/or suicide	

At least one core and four other symptoms which are present for all or most of the day every day, or nearly every day for more than 2 weeks. Must cause significant distress or impairment. Must not be due directly to the medication or general medical condition and must not be accounted for by bereavement. Advised to ignore physical symptoms in physical illness.

It is important to identify depression for the following reasons:

- more than 80% respond to treatment;
- leads to social withdrawal;
- prevents patient from completing unfinished business;
- untreated depression impacts other symptoms;
- symptoms can be worse than the illness itself.

Good practice requires all patients to be assessed for depression (NHS Lothian, 2010) as it is consistently and strongly associated with poor quality of life. The most widely accepted tool for diagnosing depression is the Diagnostic and Statistical Manual1V Classification of Disorders (DSM 1V) (American Psychiatric Association, 1994) details of which are shown in Box 10.8.

Although the DSMIV is effective in diagnosing depression, it is less effective at diagnosing depression in physical illness. There are a number of formal screening tools used to assess depression in patients receiving palliative care, some are shown in Table 10.1. There is, however,

Table 10.1 Examples of depression assessment tools.

Tool	Comment
Single question – are you depressed? (Chockinov *et al.*, 1997)	Simple and short; excellent selectivity and sensitivity in original study with cancer patients but possible different responses with different patient populations or cultural backgrounds.
Hospital Anxiety and Depression Scale (HADS) (Zigmond and Snaith, 1983)	Looks at anxiety and depression, focussing on psychological symptoms only. Validated in UK palliative care population and has similar selectivity/specificity/positive predictive value to EPDS.
Edinburgh Post Natal Depression Scale (EPDS) (Lloyd-Williams, 2000)	Short, psychological symptoms. Includes questions about suicide and self harm. Validated in UK palliative care population. Reasonably selectivity and specificity and positive predictive value.
Brief Edinburgh Scale (Lloyd-Williams *et al.* 2007)	Shortened form of the Edinburgh Post Natal Depression Scale, shown to be sensitive when used with palliative care patients.

Box 10.9 Predisposing factors to depression/anxiety

Organic mental disorders
Poorly controlled physical symptoms
Poor relationship and communication between staff and patient
Past history of mood disorders – personal or family
History of substance misuse e.g. alcohol or drug
Personality traits or lifestyle increasing susceptibility – early life time experiences, social circumstances
Lack of family and social support
Family history and genetic factors
Gender – female:male ratio 2:1
Age
Perceived inadequacy of information
Number and severity of concerns
Poor resolution of concerns
Diagnosis – oropharyngeal, pancreatic, breast and lung cancers.

Adapted from Lloyd-Williams; Parles and Maguire, 1996; Barraclough 1997 and NHS Lothian, 2010

a lack of consensus as to their benefits. Rather than using complicated tools there is some evidence that just asking patient if they feel depressed is often most effective (Chochinov *et al.*, 1997).

Patients need to be assessed carefully for previous history of anxiety, depression, alcohol and drug use in addition to previous reactions to difficult situations. Previous and current treatment should be noted. Potential trigger situations or thoughts should be identified and the presence of dread, insomnia, diaphoresis, dyspnoea and muscle tension reported (Stoklosa *et al.*, 2007). Box 10.9 lists the predisposing factors for developing depression or anxiety.

Management and treatment of anxiety and depression

Management depends on the severity of the symptoms. Treatment can significantly improve the patient's quality of life and is effective in palliative care (NHS Lothian, 2010). Mild depression and anxiety may respond well to good psychological support and effective control of physical symptoms. It may also be appropriate to attend to spiritual distress or to, refer to appropriate members of the multi-disciplinary team for interventions such as cognitive behavioural therapy, (NHS Lothian, 2010). When necessary, anxiolytics and antidepressants may need to be prescribed, examples of which are shown in Table 10.2.

Non-pharmacological treatments have also been found to be effective. These include aromatherapy (35%) counselling (8%) and herbal medication St John's Wort (3%) (Lawrie *et al.*, 2004).

Table 10.2 Examples of anxiolytic and antidepressant medication.

Group	Examples
Selective serotonin reuptake inhibitors (SSRIs)	For example, Sertraline, Citaloprim, Fluoxetine
Tricyclic antidepressants	For example, Amitryptilline, Lofepramine
Psychostimulants (6%)	
For doses and side effects please see the British National Formulary	

Sexuality

Although sexuality is a nebulous concept, attempts at formal definition are shown in Fact Box 10.4. Encompassing more than just sexual contact and intercourse (Cleary *et al.*, 2013), it includes how we feel about ourselves as male or female, the way we communicate (both verbally and non verbally) to those around us and how comfortable we are with ourselves (Wilmoth, 2013). We express sexuality in how we dress and in our relationships with others (Taylor and Davis, 2006). Sexuality is intrinsic to a person's sense of self, relating to one's need for closeness, touch, caring pleasure, relationships with others and forms part of our identity throughout life (Bauer *et al.*, 2007). Katz (2005) recognises that sexuality is a part of normal life for most people and as such it is an important aspect of quality of life.

The WHO (2006) working definition of sexuality is:

> …a central aspect of being human throughout life encompasses sex, gender identities and roles, sexual orientation, eroticism, pleasure, intimacy and reproduction. Sexuality is experienced and expressed in thoughts, fantasies, desires, beliefs, attitudes, values, behaviours, practices, roles and relationships. While sexuality can include all of these dimensions, not all of them are always experienced or expressed. Sexuality is influenced by the interaction of biological, psychological, social, economic, political, cultural, legal, historical, religious and spiritual factors.

Fact Box 10.4

Definitions of sexuality

Sexuality is a complex issue and is much more than a focus on the genital nature of sex. It involves the whole experience of self as a man or woman, including relationships with others, feelings about oneself and the physiological functioning of the body. It includes self esteem and the roles that we take on or have been given. (Griffiths, 2009)

Sexuality encompasses mind body and spirit (Tierney, 2008)

Sexuality is whatever it means to the patient (Cagle and Bolte, 2009)

Sexuality does not end with the diagnosis or progression of a life-threatening illness. Illness or the consequences of treatment may complicate the patient's social and sexual life, with the potential to diminish their self-esteem, self concept, sense of attractiveness, relationships and sexual functioning (Higgins *et al.*, 2006). It is, however, at these times, according to Wilmoth (2013), that the need for sexuality and intimacy may become even more important as a way of reaffirming connections with others, feelings of being alive and a sense of being wanted. The importance of physical expression may change during the course of an illness with greater emphasis on verbal interactions, close body contact, 'meaningful' eye contact, all leading to a greater sense of emotional connectedness (Lemiuex *et al.*, 2007). Nurses are in a unique position to help patients and families by facilitating discussion about sexual issues (Higgins *et al.*, 2006).

Activity 10.4

Consider your answers to the following questions which are based on the work of Hordern and Street (2007a).

What does sexuality mean to you? What factors influence your personal meaning of sexuality? Think of 5 ways in which you express your sexuality.

Have you ever asked a patient how the treatment/disease/illness has impacted on the intimate areas of their lives?

If you have, what was it like?

How did you feel at the time and what prompted you to do?

If you haven't, can you think back on a patient you have looked after when it might have been appropriate to do so?

Three main factors have been found to explain why sexuality and sexual expression are not addressed properly or may be totally ignored:

1. **Symptoms**
   If symptoms which impact sexuality are dominating the patient's life then sexuality may not be an immediate priority and so is not attended to. Symptoms affecting sexuality include: fatigue, pain, neutropenia and thrombocytopenia, dyspnoea, incontinence, mobility issues, decreased body image and self esteem, anxiety, depression and sexual dysfunction.
2. **Institutional barriers**
   These include lack of privacy, shared rooms, intrusion by staff and visitors, bed size, and uninviting visiting spaces. Even within the home, necessary equipment and visits by health care staff can be intrusive and depersonalising.
3. **Attitudes of health care professionals**
   Of the three main reasons why sexuality is not addressed, perhaps the most important is the attitude of HCPs. Patients want this important aspect addressed (Lemieux *et al.*, 2004) yet assume that if the topic hadn't been raised by the HCPs caring for them then the issue is not important (Redelman, 2008; Ussher *et al.*, 2013). They are often searching for practical strategies and emotional support to help them come to terms with their altered sense of sexuality. Reasons why HCPs are so reluctant to address the topic of sexuality are summarised in Box 10.10.

Box 10.10 Reasons why health care professionals are reluctant to raise issues of sexuality

- boundary issues, for example, fear of patient and carer reactions, causing offense, being intrusive or inappropriate, embarrassment for themselves and the patient;
- insufficient or inadequate knowledge and skills;
- uncomfortable and anxious about discussing sexuality with people different from themselves in terms of age, sexual orientation, ethnicity or ability;
- fear of opening up 'Pandora's Box';
- not knowing where or how to start;
- presence of partner or a third person;
- assumptions that dealing with sexuality is the responsibility of someone else;
- sexual issues are seen as unimportant compared with the struggle to overcome disease and cope with treatment;
- difficulty in including sexuality in holistic care;
- concern about what other colleagues might think;
- personal discomfort in discussing sexuality;
- lack of knowledge about sexual problems and impact of the disease or treatment;
- time/privacy constraints.

Krebs, 2008; Redelman, 2008; Horden *et al.*, 2009; Blagbrough, 2010

HCPs are prevented from talking about sexuality because of structural constraints and lack of education but also feelings of personal vulnerability and uncertainty even when they think patients have these concerns. Rather than trusting their communication skills or engaging in a reflexive communication process, they disguise their own feelings of uncertainty and vulnerability and make assumptions about the needs of patients (Hordern and Street, 2007b).

Activity 10.5

Try and think of some of the reasons why you may struggle or find it challenging to communicate with patients about sexuality.

What strategies could you use to help recognise the assumptions you bring to clinical practice?

Assessing sexuality

Nurses often do not assess sexuality fully because they perceive it in terms of sex and sexual function only, but holistic care is only provided when nurses recognise and acknowledge the importance of sexuality in their patients' lives (Mick, 2007; Ussher *et al.*, 2013). Sexual assessment should be undertaken sooner rather than later, and may be easier to complete if we consider it in terms of how concerns about issues such as body image, feelings of femininity/masculinity, roles and responsibilities within the family affect quality of life.

Generating an attitude and climate in which the patient feels free to express and discuss his or her concerns is perhaps the most important starting point (Higgins *et al.*, 2006). It is, however, also important for nurses to recognise that not everyone will want to discuss their concerns and that the patient is not under any pressure to respond to questions they don't want to answer (Higgins *et al.*, 2006). An example of how to start this conversation is given in Box 10.11.

Having begun the assessment it is important to maintain the momentum. Questions that could be used to develop the assessment are shown in Box 10.12. Box 10.13 shows examples of gentle probing questions that can be used to explore each aspect in more detail.

The assessments always need to be done sensitively, responding to the patient's readiness to discuss the issue further. Sometimes, however, it is the patient who gives us the cues that they want to talk. A cue is a clear indication that someone wants to talk and gives us opportunities to facilitate that exploration and discussion (Hargie and Dickson, 2004). We need to

Box 10.11 Starting an assessment about sexuality

I want to ask you some questions which you might feel are very personal. They relate to your body image and relationships. If you feel uncomfortable about anything it is OK not to answer.

Box 10.12 Questions to consider in assessing the impact of disease on the patient's sexuality

How has the illness changed the way you feel about yourself?

How has the diagnosis/illness/treatment affected your role as a wife/husband/parent?

How has the diagnosis/illness/treatment affected the way you feel about yourself as a man/woman?

In what ways has your condition/illness/treatment affected the way you express your sexuality?

What impact has the diagnosis/treatment/illness had on your sexual functioning?

Other people I've spoken to, have told me in similar circumstances, that the physical parts of their relationships/their self esteem/their body image has been affected by the illness. Would you like to discuss this?

It must be hard to feel good about yourself after all you've been through. How has the illness affected your relationship with ……?

Some people get frustrated by the lack of private time with their significant other. How about you?

listen and respond to these cues as these are often an indication that the patient is testing out the water to see if it is alright to talk about these issues (Higgins *et al.*, 2006). Examples of cues are shown in Box 10.14.

Many people want to grieve for the loss of sexuality, closeness and it is the nurse's role to help them tell their story. They may well talk about their loneliness, feelings of sadness, loss of intimacy, altered body image and future potential (Higgins *et al.*, 2006). Understanding sexuality from the patient's perceptions of their body image, family roles and functions, relationships and sexual function can help nurses improve their assessment of real or potential alterations in sexuality (Mick, 2007). It is worth remembering that couples are more likely to be looking for help and support in their relationships than technical advice or sex therapy.

To engage in these discussions successfully, we must first be willing to do so. We must develop a non- judgemental approach and be aware of any assumptions we may make about sexual orientation or the likelihood of the patient engaging in sexual activity. For example, a question to a female patient such as 'How does your boyfriend/husband feel about your illness?' assumes that the patient is in a heterosexual relationship. A patient's age itself is not an indicator of whether someone is sexually active, so we must avoid making ageist assumptions.

Assessing sexuality should be a routine part of our care (Ussher *et al.*, 2013) and the more we do it, the more natural such conversations seem and patients will sense that the questions are simply our routine with everyone.

Formal models provide us with a framework to guide practice and to structure our assessment (Higgins *et al.*, 2006). One such model relating to assessment of sexuality is the PLISSIT model (Annon, 1976) shown in Table 10.3.

All nurses should be able to give 'permission' and also provide limited information regarding sexuality and when nurses fail to meet these responsibilities, patients are given a disservice which has the potential to negatively affect their health and well being (Odey, 2009). Another model, the BETTER model (Mick *et al.*, 2004) is also useful in guiding an assessment of sexuality and involves the nurse being prepared to bring up the subject to make patients feel that they can express their concerns at any time. Nurses may be required to provide information about the effects of treatment on aspects of sexuality. Discussing sexuality may be considered a significant barrier for us to overcome and Mick (2007) offers us strategies to help which are shown in Box 10.15.

Box 10.13 Questions to facilitate further discussion

Tell me more about it?

What do you think might help?

What makes it better? What makes it worse?

How would you and X normally deal with issues?

Box 10.14 Examples of cues

'Looking like this, I can't bear for her to touch me'

'Everything that made me feel like a woman is missing now'

'We used to enjoy cuddling up on the settee to watch a film'

Table 10.3 PLISSIT model (Annon, 1976).

PLISSIT
P = Permission – these represent the actions taken by the nurse to let the patient and their partner know that sexuality and sexual issues are a legitimate aspect of nursing care. It can include routine questions asked through assessment or more specific ones related to the illness/disease.
LI = Limited information – this involves sharing information regarding the effects of the disease or treatment.
SS = Specific suggestions – this stage requires specialist knowledge.
IT = Intensive therapy – usually involves referral to a qualified psychotherapist or sex counsellor.
Reproduced with permission from the American Association of Sexuality Educators, Counselors and Therapists

Box 10.15 Strategies to help improve sexuality assessment (Mick, 2007)

- Understand sexuality – *see it wider than just sex and sexual function.*
- Provide information – *whatever is relevant.*
- Address causes of discomfort – *overcome by developing a wider concept of sexuality.*
- Be an objective listener – *remain objective and non judgemental when listening to patients.*
- Perform independent assessments – *to establish any issues.*
- Use practice standards – *NMC (2010).*
- Ask broad questions – *for example, how their illness affects their role in the family.*
- Avoid making assumptions – *own beliefs about sexuality and illness, age etc.*
- Learn about sexuality – *self explanatory.*
- Encourage questions – *about anything.*

Psychological care

Although the manifestations of psychological distress cannot be controlled in the same way as physical pain, neglecting to address these may adversely impact on the well being of the patient and their significant others (Amoah, 2011). The principles of psychological management are shown in Box 10.16 and the nurse's role is to assess and communicate (listen, observe, question) often using courage to act on the findings.

Achieving effective psychological care is both challenging and complex. It involves the sensitive use of effective communication skills, accurate assessment and sometimes medication to help reduce levels of distress. Other psychosocial techniques, however, are also available and are shown in Box 10.17. These may require the involvement of many members of the multi-disciplinary team.

Box 10.16 Principles of psychological management

- The sensitive breaking or telling of bad news.
- Providing information in accordance with the patient's wishes and at their pace.
- Permitting and encouraging expressions of emotions.
- Clarification of concerns and problems.
- Involving patients in decision making.
- Setting realistic and achievable goals.
- Co-ordinating appropriate packages of nursing, social and medical care.
- Ensuring continuity of care.

Box 10.17 Psychosocial techniques

- Giving relevant information in a way that the patient can understand, at a pace the patient finds acceptable and in a way the patient finds helpful.
- Encourage relaxation – deep breathing, relaxation tapes.
- Financial benefits – Ensuring the patient is receiving all financial help available.
- Cognitive behavioural therapy.
- Hypnosis.
- Acupuncture.
- Aromatherapy/massage.
- Guided imagery.
- Positive Distraction.
- Group discussions and support.
- Music therapy.
- Art therapy.
- Creative writing.
- Meditation.

Good psychological care is so important in palliative care and involves a close working relationship between HCPs and patients. Maguire (1985) found that whilst 1 in 4 patients failed to disclose problems spontaneously, HCPs in turn were reluctant to raise psychological concerns. The reasons for this are shown in Box 10.18.

Forrest (1983) found that HCPs including nurses, become adept at developing strategies to prevent patients from revealing their concerns. These are shown in Box 10.19.

Activity 10.6

Spend a few moments thinking about your practice and try and identify occasions when you might have used some of the strategies listed in Box 10.19. What were your reasons? How did it make you feel and how do you think it made the patient feel?

Box 10.18 Reasons why psychological needs remain hidden

Reasons patients fail to disclose	Reason HCPS don't raise issues
Perceived HCP as being too busy	Fear of upsetting patient
Believed HCPs are primarily concerned with physical aspects of care	Fear of causing more harm than good
Don't want to burden HCPs with their worries	Fear of prompting unanswerable or difficult questions
Don't want to complain because their treatment depends on HCPs	Fear of saying the wrong thing
Think their worries are silly or trivial	Inability to handle the emotions involved
Fear they won't be able to cope if they start talking about issues	Unable to do anything about it so why ask?
Fear they may cry or break down or lose control	Not knowing enough to answer the questions
Don't have the words to explain how they feel	Not my job!!
Anxious that their worst fears may be confirmed	

Box 10.19 Strategies to prevent patients disclosing their concerns (Forrest 1983)

Normalising/stereotyping comments – *'Everybody feels like that'; 'What do you expect?'*

Premature/false reassurance – *Jumping in to reassure before fully understanding the issue*

Inappropriate advice.

Closed/leading or multiple questions – *'How are you today? How did you sleep? What would you like for breakfast? You don't want eggs, do you?'*

Physically focussed – *keeping all questions and conversations focussed on physical issues.*

Passing the buck – *'I'll get the doctor or the priest to come and talk to you?'*

Disapproving/disagreeing – *Challenging in effect what the patient has said.*

Defending – *The attitudes, comments or actions of colleagues or family/friends.*

Changing the topic/ignoring/selective attention to cues.

Change of focus to the relative.

Jollying along – *'You'll feel better after lunch.'*

Personal chit chat – *Nurses talking to each other rather than the patient.*

Why is it so difficult to ask questions to assess psychological issue? Sometimes it could be because we find the words, subjects or ideas socially or culturally unacceptable, resulting in us feeling very uncomfortable. We may fear that we will be unable to help or that we will upset the patient. Or it could be that we are frightened that if we raise a subject, that might lead to a problem. We need to think of different ways of phrasing questions, choosing wording which we are comfortable with and then rehearse and practice so that it sounds natural.

Psychological care is not an optional extra. Indeed, NICE (2004) guidelines require us to improve psychological care through regular assessment and psychological support, where necessary. NICE (2004) identifies the four levels of intervention shown in the following fact Box.

Fact Box 10.5

NICE levels of psychological intervention

Level 1	Interventions
Recognition of psychological distress, competent to avoid causing harm, know limitations and know when to refer. Applicable for all staff	Communication with honesty, compassion, dignity and respect Establish and maintain relationships Information
Level 2	**Interventions**
Assessment at key points, diagnosis, treatment episode, end of treatment or recurrence. Assess impact on daily life, mood relationships, work, communication and listening skills, trust. Problems identified at this level maybe resolved if not – refer on. HCP trained to screen.	Simple psychological techniques – problem solving Trained and supervised HCP – could be a Clinical Nurse Specialist
Level 3	**Interventions**
Trained and accredited HCP Differentiate between moderate and sever problems Refer on	Specific psychological therapies Mild to moderate anxiety Treatment anxiety, relationship spirituality
Level 4	**Interventions**
Specialist psychological services; complex problems, co-ordination of care, emergency services, close working relationships with other teams Information transfer process	Psychosocial techniques Promote and improve coping

Reproduced with permission from National Institute for Clinical Excellence (2004) Adapted from '*Improving Supportive and Palliative Care for Adults with Cancer*. London: NICE. Available from http://guidance.nice.org.uk

Conclusion

The DH (2008) and NICE (2004) identify open and honest communication as key to effective planning and delivery of palliative care. Nowhere is this more important than in addressing psychological needs. Lack of adequate communication may heighten distress and undermine adjustment to the changes in the illness experience of patients and their significant others (Amoah, 2011). Some elements of good pastoral communication that can relieve patients' anxiety are the ability to generate an assuring presence, active listening, validating emotions and empathising (Amoah, 2011). These are skills that all nurses need and we are ideally placed to use them with patients receiving palliative care.

Glossary

Acupuncture	A component of traditional Chinese Medicine which consists of a collection of procedures involving penetrating the skin with fine needles to stimulate certain points on the body.
Acute traumatic stress disorder	Alternative name for post traumatic distress disorder; occurs after a traumatic life event and is characterised by sensations such as anxiety, numbness, flashbacks.
Adjustment disorder	Occurs within three months of a major stressor, causing considerable distress and impairment with function.
Anger	A normal emotion which involves a strong uncomfortable response to perceived provocations.
Anorexia	A reduced appetite.
Anti anxiolytics	A group of medications given to combat anxiety.
Anti depressants	A group of medications given to combat depression.
Anxiety	A state of apprehension and fear leading to a perception of a threat to oneself.
Aromatherapy	A form of complimentary therapy that uses plant essential oils for the purpose of altering a person's mood, cognitive function or health.
Autonomic	Relates to part of the peripheral nervous system that acts as a control below the level of consciousness, controlling visceral functions.
Cognitive behavioural therapy	A psychotherapeutic approach that uses a number of goal-orientated, explicit systematic procedures to address dysfunctional emotions, maladaptive behaviours or thoughts.
Cue	A clear indication that someone wants to talk about something and gives the listener the opportunity to raise the subject.

Cultural needs	Those needs that arise from a patient's culture.
Depression	A prolonged low mood affecting the ability to carry out day to day activities.
Delusions	A strong conviction that something is true despite evidence to the contrary
Diaphoresis	Excessive sweating.
Diurnal variation	Becoming an 'owl' rather than a 'lark'.
Dyspnoea	Shortness of breath.
Early morning waking	Waking in the early hours of the morning, a symptom often associated with depression.
Euthanasia	The practice of intentionally ending a life in order to relieve suffering.
Existential	Concerns related to the meaning of human existence.
Fatigue	A subjective feeling of tiredness.
Generalised anxiety disorder	Characterised by pervasive and excessive anxiety and worry about events for many days, for a period of at least six months.
Guided imagery	With the help of a therapist, using the imagination to help with healing or reducing stress.
Hallucination	A perception mimicking a real perception without an apparent stimulus.
Holistic care	Care based on the belief that the patient is more than a sum of their parts; recognises the importance of the physical, psychological, social and spiritual dimensions.
Hypnosis	A special psychological state, resembling sleep but marked by the patient functioning at a level of awareness different from the ordinary conscious state.
Indecisiveness	The inability to make decisions, often a symptom of anxiety and depression.
Insomnia	The inability to fall asleep or stay asleep as long as desired.
Intractable pain	Chronic pain from which it is difficult to get relief.
Libido	The patient's desire for sex or sexual activity.
Meditation	A broad variety of practices in which the patient trains mind in order to promote relaxation.

Mental health	A level of psychological well being or an absence of a mental disorder.
Music therapy	The clinical and evidence based use of music interventions to accomplish patients' goals within a therapeutic relationship.
Person centred care	Care which places the patient at its centre.
Post traumatic stress disorder	Alternative name for acute traumatic distress disorder; occurs after a traumatic life event and is characterised by sensations such as anxiety, numbness, flashbacks.
Psychological distress	A multi-factorial unpleasant emotional experience which may interfere with one's ability to cope.
Psychomotor slowing	The slowing down of the thought process and a reduction of physical movements.
Sadness	An emotional pain associated with feelings of disadvantage, loss, despair, helplessness and sorrow.
Severe adjustment reaction	A severe reaction in response to bad news.
Sex therapy	The treatment of sexual dysfunction, including those of physical or psychological origin.
Social withdrawal	Removing oneself from friends and activities; often symptomatic of anxiety and depression.
Somatic symptoms	Related to physical symptoms.
Spiritual distress	A disturbance of a person's belief system.
Stigma	Attached to a person who is considered 'different' in some way from the rest of society.
Sympathy	A feeling, concern and reaction to the distress or need of another person.

Patient scenarios

Keith Jones is a 78-year-old married man who has lived with COPD for the past 20 years. Keith has always managed his illness well with the support of the local chronic conditions nurse. His breathlessness has been getting steadily worse, exacerbated by several chest infections over the recent winter months. Following some frank discussions with his nurse Keith has come to realise that his prognosis is now significantly shorter. Along with his breathlessness he is experiencing difficulties in sleeping and concentrating, he has noticed that his mouth is drier than normal and that he is often pre-occupied.

Activity 10.7

What do you think is causing these symptoms?

How would you assess Keith?

What nursing care do you think would be appropriate?

Answer:

The symptoms are caused by increased anxiety and possibly depression in response to worsening symptoms and altered prognosis and concerns about how his wife will manage once he is dead.

Assess using HAD score to differentiate between anxiety and depression.

Nursing care will include

effective communication using open questions and picking up on cues;
giving Keith time to explore issues and express his concerns;
referral to GP for anxiolytics or anti depressants (depending on HAD score).

References

Agrawal M; Danis M; (2002) End-of-life care for terminally ill participants in clinical research. *Journal of Palliative Medicine.* 5(5): 729–37.

American Psychiatric Association (1994) *Diagnostic and Statistical Manual of Mental Disorders DSM-IV.* Washington D.C.: American Psychiatric Association.

Amoah, C.F. (2011) The central importance of spirituality in palliative care. *International Journal of Nursing.* 17(7): 353–358.

Annon, J. (1976) The PLISSIT model: a proposed conceptual scheme for the behavioural treatment of sexual problems. *Journal of Sex Education Therapy.* 2(2): 1–15.

Barraclough, J. (1997) ABC of palliative care: Depression, anxiety and confusion. *British Journal of Medicine.* 315(7119): 1365–1368.

Bauer, M., McAuliffe, L. and Nay, R. (2007) Sexuality, health care and the older person: an overview of the literature. *International Journal of Older People Nursing.* 2: 63–68.

Blagbrough, J. (2010) Importance of sexual needs assessment in palliative care. *Nursing Standard.* 24(52): 35–39.

Cagle, J.G. and Bolte, S. (2009) sexuality and life threatening illness: implications for social work and palliative care. *Health and Social Work.* 34(3): 223–233.

Chochinov, H., Wilson, K., Enns, M. and Lander, S. (1997) Are you depressed? Screening for depression in the terminally ill. *American Journal of Psychiatry* 154: 674–676.

Cleary, V., Hegarty, J. and McCarthy, G. (2013) How a diagnosis of gynaecological cancer affects women's sexuality. *Cancer Nursing Practice.* 12(1): 32–35.

Department of Health (2008) *End of Life Care Strategy: Promoting High Quality Care For Adults at the End of Their Life. London*: Department of Health.

Dudgeon, D., King, S., Howell, D., Green, E., Gilbert, J., Hughes, E., Lalonde, B., Angus, H. and Sawka, C. (2012) Cancer Care Ontario's experience with implementation of routine physical and psychological distress screening. *Psycho-Oncology.* 21: 357–364.

Griffith, R.W. (2009) *Sex & Aging Fact Sheet for Women* Available at www.healthandage.com/sex-and-aging-fact-sheet-for-women [accessed 17 February 2014].

Hargie, O. and Dickson, D. (2004) *Skilled Interpersonal Communication: Research, Theory and Practice* 4th edn. London: Routledge, Taylor & Francis.

Higgins, A., Barker, P. and Begley, C.M. (2006) Sexuality: The challenge to espoused holistic care. *International Journal of Nursing Practice.* 12: 345–351.

Hordern, A. J. and Street, A.F. (2007a) Let's talk about sex: Risky business for cancer and palliative care clinicians. *Contemporary Nurse.* 27 (1): 49–60.

Hordern, A.J. and Street, A.F. (2007b) Constructions of sexuality and intimacy after cancer: patient and health professionals perspectives. *Social Science and Medicine.* 64: 1704–1718.

Katz, A. (2005) The sounds of silence: sexuality information for cancer patients. *Journal of Clinical Oncology.* 1 (1): 238–241.

Krebs, L.U. (2008) Sexual assessment in cancer care: concepts, methods and strategies for success. *Seminars in Oncology Nursing.* 24(2): 80–90.

International Association for the Study of Pain (2009) *Total Cancer Pain* Available at http://www.iaspain.org/AM/Template.cfm?Section=Fact_Sheets1&Template=/CM/ContentDisplay.cfm&ContentID=8705 [accessed 17 February 2014].

Lawrie, I., Lloyd-Williams, M. and Taylor, F. (2004) How do palliative medicine physicians assess and manage depression. *Palliative Medicine.* 18(3): 234–238.

Lemieux, L., Kaiser, S., Pereira, J. and Meadows, L. (2004) Sexuality in palliative care: patients perspectives. *Palliative Medicine* 18(7): 630–637.

Lloyd-Williams, M. (2000) Difficulties in diagnosing and treating depression in the terminally ill cancer patient. *Postgraduate Medical Journal.* 76(899): 555–8.

Lloyd-Williams, M. (2003) Screening for depression in palliative care In Lloyd-Williams, M. (ed) *Psychosocial issues in palliative care.* Oxford: Oxford University Press Chapter 7.

Lloyd-Williams, M., Sheils, C. and Dowrick, C. (2007) The development of the Brief Edinburgh Depression Scale (BEDS) to screen for depression in patients with advanced cancer. *Journal of Affective Disorders* 99: 259–264.

Macleod, S. (2007) *The Psychiatry of Palliative Medicine: The Dying Mind.* Oxford: Radcliffe Publishers.

Mick, J. (2007) Sexuality assessment: 10 strategies for improvement. *Clinical Journal of Oncology Nursing.* 11(5): 671–675.

Mick, J., Hughes, M. and Cohen, M.Z. (2004) Using the BETTER model to assess sexuality. *Clinical Journal of Oncology Nursing.* 8: 84–86.

National Comprehensive Cancer Network (2010) *Clinical Guidelines in Oncology – Distress Management* Available at www.nccn.org/professionals/physician_gls/f_guidelines.asp [accessed 17 February 2014].

NICE (2004) *Guidance on Cancer: Improving Supportive and Palliative Care for Adults with Cancer.* London: Spiritual Support Services NICE Available at http://www.nice.org.uk/nicemedia/pdf/csgspman-ual.pdf [accessed 17 February 2014].

National Council of Hospice and Specialist Palliative Care Services (1997) *Feeling Better: Psychological Care in specialist Palliative Care* Occasional paper no 13 London NCPSPCS

Nursing and Midwifery Council (2010) *Standards for preregistration education.* London: Nursing and Midwifery Council.

Odey, K. (2009) Legitimizing patient sexuality and sexual health to provide holistic care. *Gastointestinal Nursing* 7(8): 43–47.

Redelman, M. (2008) Is there a place for sexuality in the holistic care of patients in the palliative care phase of life?. *American Journal of Hospital Palliative Medicine* 25 (5): 366–371.

Stoklosa, J., Patterson, K., Rosielle, D. and Arnold, R. (2007) *Anxiety in Palliative Care – Causes and Diagnosis.* Fast Facts and Concepts. 186 Available at http://www.eperc.mcw.edu/EPERC/FastFactsIndex/ff_186.htm [accessed 24 February 2014].

Taylor, B. and Davis, S. (2006) Using the extended PLISSIT model to address sexual health care needs. *Nursing Standard* 21 (11): 35–40.

Tierney, D.K. (2008) Sexuality assessment in cancer care *Seminars in Oncology Nursing.* 24(92): 80–90.

Ussher, J.; Perz, J. and Gilbert, E. (2013) Information needs associated with changes to sexual well-being after breast cancer. *Journal of Advanced Nursing* 69 (2): 327–337.

Wilmoth, M.C. (2013) Sexuality In Lubkin, I.M. and Larsen, P.D. *Chronic Illness Impact and Interventions.* London: Jones and Bartlett Chapter 11, 289–313.

World Health Organisation (2006) Available at: http://www.who.int/reproductivehealth/topics/sexual_health/sh_definitions/en/ [accessed 17 February 2014].

Zigmond, A.S. and Snaith, R. P. (1983) The hospital and depression (HAD) scale *Acta Psychiatr Scand* 67: 361–70.

Additional reading/Useful resources

Horden, A., Grainger, M., Hegarty, S.; Jefford, M., White, V. and Sutherland, G. (2009) Discussing sexuality in the clinical setting: the impact of a brief training program for oncology health professionals to enhance communication about sexuality. *Asia-Pacific Journal of Clinical Oncology.* 5: 270–277.

Price, B. (2010) Sexuality: raising the issue with patients. *Cancer Nursing Practice* 9(5): 29–35.

11

Caring for the family

Introduction

The diagnosis of a life-threatening illness and managing its consequences affects the patient and family (Belgacem *et al.*, 2013). Zaider and Kissane (2007) identify that the family is a vital resource for these patients, with its importance increasing as the illness progresses towards its final stages. The WHO's (2013) definition of palliative care in Fact Box 11.1, clearly identifies that an integral part of the discipline is caring for families. Indeed one of the fundamental principles of palliative care is that it offers a support system to help the family cope during the patient's illness and into their own bereavement (Saunders, 2006). Considered as part of the 'unit of care' within palliative care, the family plays multiple roles. On the one hand, as receivers of care, they can be thought of as 'patients' whilst on the other hand, as deliverers of care they can be

Fact Box 11.1

Definition of palliative care (WHO, 2013)

Palliative care improves the quality of life of patients and families who face life-threatening illness, by providing pain and symptom relief, spiritual and psychosocial support from diagnosis to the end of life and bereavement.

Fundamentals of Palliative Care for Student Nurses, First Edition. Megan Rosser and Helen C. Walsh.

Companion website: www.wiley.com/go/rosser_walsh/fundamentals_of_palliative_care

considered to be 'staff' (Munroe and Oliviere, 2009). Patients want to be assured that their families and carers will receive support during their illness (NICE, 2004).

Although caring for the family is an important and recognised role in palliative care, it is not exactly clear what it is or how it's done (Smith and Skilbeck, 2008). This chapter attempts to add some clarity to this, through exploring the challenges for families in caring for loved ones. It begins by exploring what is meant by the term 'family', before considering the role of the family in caring. The effects that caring has on the family and factors which influence their abilities to cope are considered. The needs of families are identified and good practice discussed.

Learning outcomes

By the end of this chapter you should be able to

- define what we mean by the term 'family';
- discuss the role of the family in caring for the patient;
- recognise the effects of caring and those factors which enable families to cope;
- identify the needs of family;
- discuss good practice in relation to caring for the family.

Defining the family

One of the first challenges of caring for the family is recognising who makes up 'the family' (Smith, 2001). As a consequence of considerable changes within society the term 'family' is more difficult to define nowadays. Families have become smaller and more scattered, the extended family is less important and the nuclear family less clearly identifiable with the number of second families, step families and same sex families increasing. The family is becoming more diverse and, therefore, more difficult to define. While considerably dated, Bell and Wright (1994) offer a helpful definition for 'family' shown in Fact Box 11.2. This definition allows flexibility and enables the family to be whoever the patient says it is (Kissane and Bloch, 2002) and can include blood relatives, friends, neighbours and other significant relationships identified by the patient.

Fact Box 11.2

Definition of family (Bell and Wright, 1994)

A family is a group of individuals who are bound by strong emotional ties, a sense of belonging and a passion for being involved in one another's lives.

Throughout this chapter, the term 'family' is used to mean biological family, informal care givers, friends or indeed anyone who matters to the patient.

It is important to identify the 'family' structure and existing support systems. Patients might find it difficult to identify who their family is and the title of a relationship does not necessarily indicate its relevance or importance. For example, the relationship with a neighbour who we see every day may be far stronger and more important than that with a sister who we see intermittently, if at all. One way of helping to establish those who are important to the patient is to develop a genogram or a family tree. An example of a genogram is shown in Figure 11.1 and this represents Peter and his family, details of which can be seen in Box 11.1.

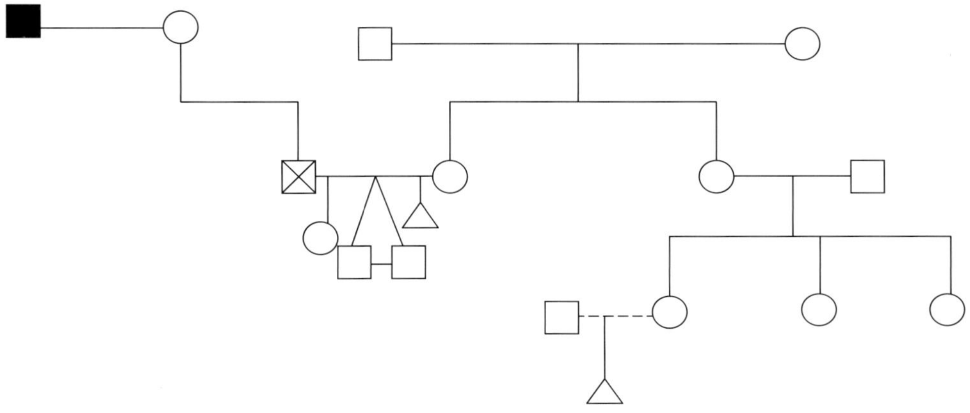

Figure 11.1 Genogram for Peter and his family.

Box 11.1 Peter and family

Peter is 35-years old and is married to Julia. They have 3 children; Sally who is 6, David and Simon who are 2-year old twins and are expecting their fourth child soon. They are both teachers who worked full time until Peter was diagnosed with lymphoma 18 months ago. They have been well supported by Will and Jenny (Julia's parents) and Jane and Alan (Peter's parents). Both sets of parents live nearby and have always been incredibly supportive since the children arrived. They have also been actively involved in supporting the family in practical and financial ways since Peter's diagnosis and his inability to work. Unfortunately, Alan had a fatal heart attack 4 weeks ago and the family is in shock. Julia has been looking to her parents for increased support both practically and emotionally.

Although Peter is an only child, Julia has a younger sister, Gill. Married to Andrew, she has three daughters, Alice who is 16, Amelia 14 and Gemma 10. Alice has been seeing Wesley for the last year and has recently discovered she is pregnant. She is determined to continue with the pregnancy. Although Gill has also been very supportive of Peter and Julia, the news of Alice's pregnancy has come as a tremendous shock, causing considerable distress within her family. Amelia has become attention seeking. Andrew is not particularly supportive of Gill, Peter and Julia. Gill has increasingly turned to Will and Jenny for help.

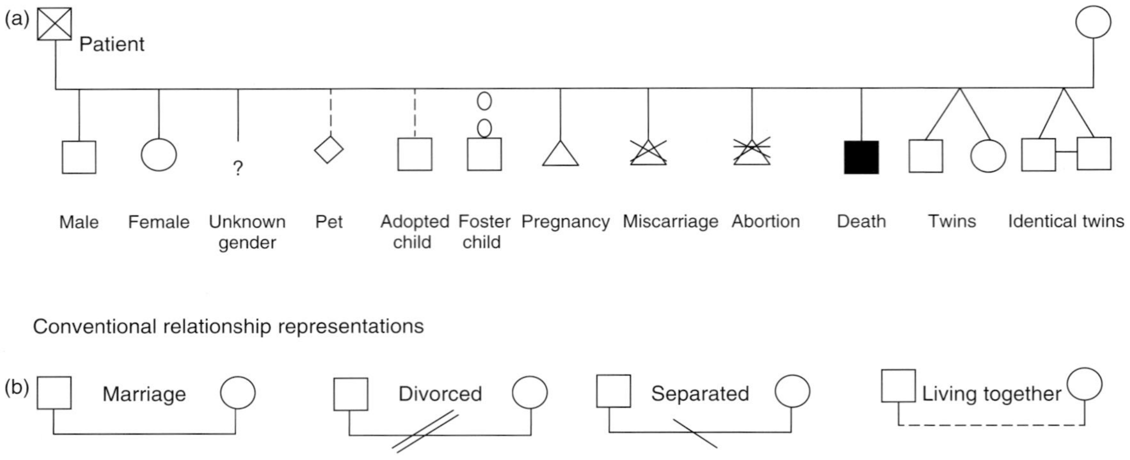

(a)
Patient
?
Male
Female
Unknown gender
Pet
Adopted child
Foster child
Pregnancy
Miscarriage
Abortion
Death
Twins
Identical twins
Conventional relationship representations
(b)
Marriage
Divorced
Separated
Living together

Figure 11.2 (a) Conventional gender symbols. (b) Conventional relationship representations.

Multiple marriages
First wife
Second wife
Third partner
Half brother

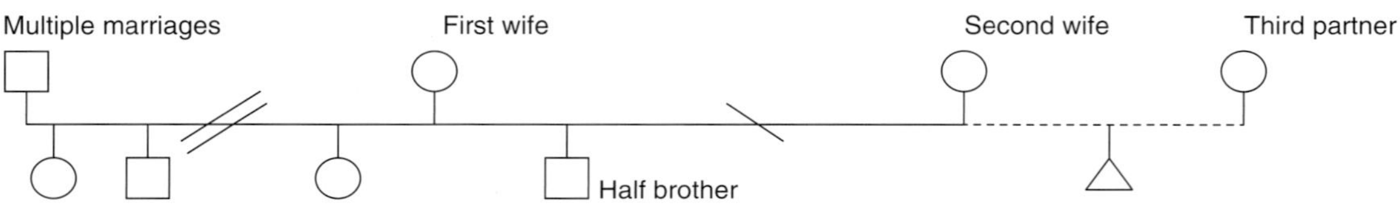

Figure 11.3 A genogram showing multiple partnerships.

Once the genogram has been constructed, additional information such as ages, occupations and so on can be added. Conventional symbols and relationship lines are shown in Figure 11.2, whilst an illustration of a genogram for multiple partners is shown in Figure 11.3.

Activity 11.1

Consider your own family and those who are close to you. Using the information in Figures 11.2 and 11.3, develop a genogram for your 'family'.

Role of the family in care giving

Family members fulfil a variety of roles whilst caring for the patient. These roles can either relate to direct or indirect care.

Direct care

Direct care involves providing simple, and in some cases complex, nursing care such as bathing, feeding, changing dressings and providing medication. Such personal tasks may well be undertaken by those closest to the patient, who may well receive companionship and emotional support during the time that they spend together. Whilst these people may also help with household chores and transport to and from medical appointments, these are often tasks that those who are not so emotionally involved are happy to help with.

Indirect care

Zaider and Kissane (2007) identify that family members

- serve as primary caretakers overseeing the patient and the care given in the community setting;
- guide provision of support from informal and formal sources;
- actively participate in decision-making, particularly if the patient can no longer be involved;
- act as proxy informants to health care professionals, giving them information on behalf of the patient.

The role of the family should not be underestimated. For example, families can either facilitate or prevent effective pain and symptom control. By ensuring that the patient takes the correct dose of medication at the correct time and accurately reporting its effects, families can ensure that health care professionals receive the information they need to manage symptoms. If families are scared of strong analgesics such as morphine or reluctant for the patient to be given sedatives, then symptom control is compromised. While Aspinal *et al.* (2002) have shown that families can act as an accurate proxy for patients in reporting the level of symptom distress, Panke and Ferrell (2005) recognise that it is also possible for them to

- over-estimate the patient's 'suffering' and distress or
- under-estimate it, in an attempt to deny that the disease is progressing.

The extent to which individual family members are involved in the patient's care depends on numerous factors including the nature of the relationship, individual experiences, age, gender and most importantly the wishes of the patient.

Effects of caring on the family

The way the family responds to the challenges of caring for someone receiving palliative care depends on numerous factors which have been highlighted in Box 11.2.

Life-threatening illness takes its toll on all members of the family; often we can see a ripple effect where something that hurts one person, acts like a wave touching other members of the family (Lee, 2010). The demands on the family, however, are not static and change in terms of the types and amounts required over the course of the illness (Smith and Skilbeck, 2008). Patients want to spend as little time as possible in hospital which can result in increasing demands on family (Belgacem *et al.*, 2013).

Box 11.2 Factors influencing the family response to serious illness

Existing perception of the disease, implications of the diagnosis, its likely trajectory and prognosis

Existing resources available to them, financial, practical and emotional

Past experiences of this disease, caring, health services

Current support available to them on physical, psychological, social, spiritual and practical levels

Outlook – could this be a positive experience or is it the last straw?

Caring for the patient can often leave family members feeling physically and mentally exhausted, resulting in them also needing to be 'looked after'. At the very basis of the care we provide to families is the need to recognise and value their contribution (Becker, 2010), encouraging other members of the health care team to do so if necessary. Failure to provide adequate support to the family can potentially result in unwanted admissions and a sense of general dissatisfaction felt by all those involved; the patient, family and the multidisciplinary team (Smith and Skilbeck, 2008). The most serious consequence is a family breakdown which may continue long after the patient has died.

It is well acknowledged that the dying patient experiences pain on a number of levels, it is also true that family members feel pain. Whilst the pain of the family is different from that of the patient, it may be as great and on occasions greater than that of the patient. The heavy burden of caring can lead to family members experiencing distress, depression and a reduction in their quality of life (Belgacem *et al.*, 2013). Box 11.3 illustrates the 'care-giver burden' which families have to cope with.

Activity 11.2

Think about a family you have been involved with where a member has received palliative care and look at the 'care giver burden' in Box 11.4. Try and identify how these apply to the family you have identified.

Influences on coping

As we have seen, the family provides care for the patient in many ways and providing that care is costly for them. It is, therefore, necessary for us to provide palliative care for the family. Recognising the family as part of the unit of care (WHO, 2013) and intervening as early as possible enables us to offer family members care, which has the potential to create and strengthen cohesion within the family thus preventing crisis and breakdown. Interventions with the family can vary from merely actively listening to what individuals within the family are saying to

Box 11.3 'Care-giver burden' (Kristjanson *et al.*, 2003; McIntyre and Lugton, 2005; Panke and Ferrell, 2005)

Altered roles and activities.

Juggling existing and new demands – work and caring.

Changing responsibilities in family.

Present situation and thoughts about the future.

Sense of helplessness.

Impact of watching 'loved one' deteriorate.

Shift in thoughts regarding meaning of life and relationships as the life of someone they love draws to a close.

Anticipated loss.

Box 11.4 Factors contributing to individuals coping with being a carer

Factors increasing abilities to cope	**Factors reducing abilities to cope**
Being able to continue with previous activities/hobbies as much as possible	The inability to continue with previous activities/hobbies
Being able to maintain hope	Feeling afraid
Receiving good levels of satisfaction with the care they give	Feeling insecure
Being able to maintain a sense of control	Feeling alone
Receiving what they identify is good support	Feeling unsupported

facilitating family therapy. The scale and level of intervention can only be identified following a comprehensive assessment of the way the individual family functions. Often various members of the multi-disciplinary palliative care team are needed to help meet the diverse family needs (Panke and Ferrell, 2005).

Robinson (1992) found that those families who are more flexible, direct, tolerant of individualism with consistent ways of communication are able to cope with taking on the caring role better. Effective care giving families are also cohesive units, where emotions are freely expressed and levels of conflict are low (Kissane and Bloch, 2002). Families are however made up of individuals who have different coping abilities when it comes to enabling them to take on the role of care giver. Those factors which help or hinder these coping abilities are shown in Box 11.4.

The needs of carers

While developing a tool to assess the needs of carers' needs, Ewing *et al.* (2012) discovered that needs fell into two distinct groups. The first group related to the support carers required enabling them to care for their loved one and the second to more direct personal care for themselves (Ewing *et al.*, 2012).

Activity 11.3

Revisit the family you thought about in Activity 11.2. What do you think their needs may have been, and try and link them to the two groups identified by Ewing *et al.* (2012). Compare your answers with those identified in Table 11.1 Carer's Needs.

Table 11.1 Carer's needs.

Practical help – this may range from help with simple household tasks such as cleaning, shopping etc to providing lifts for visiting, dog walking.
Financial help – having a family member who is ill may affect income. This could be because the patient is no longer able to work or because the carers have to stop working to care. While some employers offer sick pay, many others do not. There are also potentially many costs in looking after someone who is ill for example buying food for special diets, travelling costs for hospital appointments or visiting, prescription charges. It is therefore essential that the families are aware of the benefits available and offered help to apply for them.
Emotional support – families may face a dichotomy between wanting as much time as possible with their 'loved one', wanting death to be as far away as possible and not wanting them to 'suffer' any more. Watching someone they love go through the process of living and dying with a terminal illness results in vicarious suffering for the relatives. They need support to help them deal with these emotions.
Information – families need information to help them plan, prepare and manage the situation, although different individuals may need different information at different times. They need to know what services and resources are available locally for them. It is a challenge to know what information the family wants to know and how to give it appropriately (Smith and Skilbeck, 2008).
Spiritual support – facing this situation unavoidably raises existential questions such as 'Why?' 'What's it all about?' 'What happens afterwards?' There are no definitive answers to these questions and often the family just needs the space to ask them. Some may find comfort in their usual spiritual or religious practices, whilst others may turn away from them. Others may suddenly find comfort from formal religion in ways that they haven't before.
To be involved – families need to be given the opportunity to be involved in caring for their relative through: - giving direct care - providing emotional support - participating in decision making.

Information needs

These are a priority for the family. Those who do not receive sufficient information at the start of the patient's illness have more needs and less confidence in the healthcare system, consequently they do not cope as well as those who have had these needs met (Stetz and Hanson, 1992; Thorne and Robinson, 1988 in Kristjanson *et al.*, 2003). Families need information about the illness, how to care for the patient and how to provide comfort. While they do not necessarily need to have full medical or pharmacological explanation about the various treatments and medications, they do need to know about possible side effects and what to do if these arise. Knowing what to expect as the disease progresses is vital information, but this needs to be given at an appropriate time and pace. Too much too soon could well cause unnecessary anxiety and worry. The family also need to know how to recognise changes in the patient's condition and what to do and whom to contact if something happens. They may need help to facilitate effective communication within the family and how to keep people informed as to what is happening, for example young children or elderly parents.

Providing the family with information helps them on a number of levels. Most importantly it re-introduces a sense of control and equips the family to participate in shared decision-making (Wilkes *et al.*, 200; Kristjanson *et al.*, 2003; Panke and Ferrell, 2005). Information needs to be relayed in the most appropriate way for the individual and the family. It should be simple and as specific as possible. Information may be factual and practical addressing education needs relating to the illness, medications and the practicalities of nursing someone. The carer must be told what symptoms the patient is likely to experience. When family members don't know what is happening, they can become frightened and upset. Watching someone they love die is stressful enough, but if they know what could happen and what they can do if it does, they can prepare themselves to deal with it (Ingleton *et al.*, 2004).

Assessing the needs of the family is not always easy and requires us to listen carefully to what is actually verbalised and also to the surrounding subtext. Ewing *et al.* (2012) developed the carer support needs assessment tool (CSNAT) which is an evidenced based, validated measure of family carers' support needs. A direct measure of support needs assesses families in the following areas: physical, practical, social, financial, psychological and spiritual, all of which are domains recommended for assessment in current policy guidelines (NICE, 2004; DoH, 2008).

Good practice

Andershed and Ternestedt (1999) concluded that there were three core themes for the family caring for a person receiving palliative care. These are:

- Knowing – sharing information about the illness diagnosis, treatment, prognosis, symptoms, what to expect, available services, financial benefits and costs (Andershed and Ternestedt, 2001).
- Being – spending time and being close to one another, able to talk about things and sharing feelings. Also time to be themselves, away from the patient and with others.
- Doing – the practical acts of caring.

Andershed and Ternestedt (1999) concluded that without 'knowing', the family were limited in the level to which they could fulfil the themes of being and doing. The challenge for us as nurses is to enable the family to 'know' and facilitate them to 'be' and 'do'.

Activity 11.4

Once again, think about a family caring for someone who has been receiving palliative care. In what ways have you helped them to know, be and do? If you haven't been in this position, try and think of ways by which you could facilitate these activities.

Nurses need to work in partnership with the families, sharing knowledge appropriately and at the right time for the individuals involved. We also need to be prepared to learn from the family, recognising them as the experts on their own individual situation (Hanson, 2003). Becker (2010) suggests that it is a good practice to assign one member of the team to work directly with the family to discover their wishes, for example, how involved in the patient's care do they want to be and what, if any, specific needs/wants they have. This provides continuity in care and also identifies a point of contact among the care team for the family and a point of reference for the care team.

It is during the assessment process that we are able to develop an impression of the family structure, their unique methods of communication and needs, whether openly acknowledged or not. Some examples of the types of questions we can ask are shown in Box 11.5. Using a genogram for the family can help as a prompt to help with this process.

Each of the questions listed in Box 11.5 can be used as a springboard to evaluate or reassess the situation. For example, *When I saw you last, you said your biggest concern was xxxxxx. How is the situation now?*

Box 11.5 Useful assessment questions for use with the family (Wright and Leahey, 2000 cited by McIntyre and Lugton, 2005)

Which of your families/ friends would you wish/ not wish us to share information with?

This helps to identify alliances and conflicts which may be actual or potential.

Within your family who do you believe is the most distressed at the moment?

This helps identify who might have the greatest support needs at the present time.

What is the single biggest challenge for the family right now?

This helps to explore the family's beliefs about illness.

What could we be doing that would be most helpful to you and the family right now?

This helps to explore their expectations of care, identifies ways of collaboration and also to prioritise needs.

What is the most burning question for you at this moment in time?

This identifies major concerns at this moment in time.

Undertaking continual reassessment is important to ensure that the family's potentially changing needs are identified and their support needs addressed. We need to remember to consider the impact of the following on the family:

- emotional impact of watching someone they love deteriorate;
- emotional and physical impact caused by the additional challenges of providing practical and nursing care;
- a reduced social life for individuals, which may also include the withdrawal from the very people who would normally provide support and this could include other family members;
- actual or potentially limited social and employment roles.

Involving the family in caring for the patient is almost a given within the community setting as without family support a patient is unlikely to be able to remain in his or her own home. It becomes challenging to continue this involvement if the patient is admitted to the hospital. Having cared for them at home the family may feel guilty that the patient has been admitted and feel they have abandoned their loved one (Belgacem *et al.*, 2013). While they may also feel intimidated to ask for their involvement in practical care to continue they may also be relieved that someone else – a professional – has taken over. The skill is to use sensitive communication skills to identify the wishes of the family, and of course the patient.

Maintaining the idea that the patient and family is the unit of care (WHO, 2013) is challenging and we may need to divide our time and care between the patient and the family. There can be potential discord if patient and families have different 'wants' or expectations, again highlighting the need for effective communication skills.

Communicating with the family

Open and sensitive communication is as necessary when communicating with the family as it is when communicating with the patient. The skills required are the same and these have been discussed in detail in Chapter 6. It might be useful to review those skills at this point.

Activity 11.5

Think about an example when you experienced good communication with the family of a patient receiving palliative care. Try and identify what factors contributed to making the communication effective.

Now think of an example when you experienced difficulties communicating with the family of a patient receiving palliative care. Try and identify what factors contributed to making the communication difficult.

If you compare your answers from Activity 11.5, you will probably find that good communication has occurred when there is openness and honesty between all those involved. It becomes more difficult when things are less open and honest. The way in which dying patients, their families and the health care professionals involved, communicate is heavily influenced by the degree to which the individuals involved, acknowledge what is happening. Glaser and Strauss (1965) describe a range of 'awareness contexts' in which the patient,

Fact Box 11.3 Awareness contexts (Glaser and Strauss, 1965)

Closed awareness – everyone involved fails to recognise the reality of the situation and ultimate prognosis. Issues cannot be discussed with honesty as no one acknowledges the true situation.

Suspicion awareness – whilst the family and health care professionals are fully aware of the prognosis, the patient has merely unconfirmed suspicions. The professionals and family may feel as though they are walking on eggshells.

Mutual pretence – everyone is fully aware of the situation but tacitly agree to pretend otherwise. No one asks relevant questions so the truth of the situation is not acknowledged or the situation discussed.

Open awareness – where everyone is fully aware of what is happening and communication about the impending death is open and honest.

family and to some extent health care professionals, may exist. These are illustrated in Fact Box 11.3.

It is clear from reading the contents of that box, that communication is much easier when open awareness exists. Even at this point, however, we have to be very sensitive to what is happening for the family and patient at any particular time. While they may be open and honest today, the pain and emotional stress of the situation may lead them to seek refuge and solace in closed awareness tomorrow. Our conversations should always be guided by the family and we should make no assumptions.

Conclusion

Families are extremely important within palliative care (Lee, 2010). While working with them can be extremely challenging, it is also extremely rewarding (Smith and Skilbeck, 2008). One of the challenges for nurses is to help the family manage the emotional aspects of caring through enabling exploration of the satisfaction that caring can bring (Hanson, 2003). As nurses, we must never forget that family carers need to be supported in their central role of caring for their loved ones at the end of life (Ewing *et al.*, 2012).

We can care for families by recognising their uniqueness and the extraordinary situation in which they find themselves. Munroe and Oliviere (2009) recognise that families are made up of ordinary people who, as a result of the illness and bereavement react, respond, adjust and achieve. Although we need to involve families in caring for their loved ones, perhaps the most effective way we can demonstrate our care of for them is in the way we care for the patient, ensuring that they are well cared for and any symptoms controlled as well as possible. As McIntyre (2002: p208) cited by McIntyre and Lugton (2005) points out:

> *'Relatives seem to need reassurance that the special status of their dying loved one will be recognised. When relatives see staff showing warmth and friendship toward the*

patient they feel greatly comforted. In such an emotional climate if relatives have to leave the patient's bedside for a spell, they are reassured that there will be someone who really cares about their relatives until they return'

Glossary

Care Support Needs Assessment Tool	An evidence based, validated measure of carers support needs.
Closed awareness	Patient family and cares all fail to recognise the reality of the situation.
Emotional pain	Occurs in response to the losses associated with the illness.
Extended family	Includes all generations of the nuclear family, for example, grandparents, great grandparents, aunts, uncles, cousins etc
Family	A group of individuals bound by strong emotional ties.
Family therapy	A branch of psychotherapy that works with families to nurture change/development and emphasises family relationships as an important factor of psychological health.
Family tree	A chart representing family relationships in conventional 'tree' structure.
Genogram	Used in medicine and social work, these are more detailed than the conventional family tree.
Life-threatening illness	A long term or chronic illness which has the potential to reduce life expectancy.
Mutual pretence	While everyone is aware of the situation there is tacit agreement that it is not discussed.
Nuclear family	A pair of adults and their children.
Open awareness	Everyone involved, including the patient is aware of what is happening and communication is open and honest.
Physical pain	Results from the damage done to tissues as a result of the disease process.
Same sex family	Where the parents are of the same sex.

Second family	One or both of the parents have children from previous relationships, with new offspring sharing the same parents.
Social pain	Results from increasing isolation as the illness advances.
Spiritual pain	Results from unanswered existential questions.
Step/blended family	One parent has children that are not related to the other parent and either one or both parents have children from another relationship.
Suspicion awareness	Those around the patient are aware of the situation but the patient has only unconfirmed suspicions.

References

Andershed, B. and Ternestedt, B. (1999) Involvement of relatives in care of the dying in different care cultures: development of a theoretical understanding. *Nursing Science Quarterly*. 12(1): 45–51.

Andershed, B. and Ternestedt, B. (2001) Development of a theoretical framework describing relatives involvement in palliative care. *Journal of Advanced Nursing*. 34(4): 55–62.

Aspinal, F., Hughes, R., Higginson, I.J., Chidgey, J., Drescher, U. and Thompson, M.A. (2002) *A user's Guide to the Palliative Care Outcome Scale*. London: Palliative Care and Policy Publications.

Becker, R. (2010) *Fundamental Aspects of Palliative Care Nursing: An Evidence-Based Handbook for Student Nurses* 2nd edn. London: Quay Books.

Belgacem, B., Auclair, C., Fedor, M.C., Brugnon, D., Blanquet, M.,Tournilhac, O., Gerbaud, L. (2013) A caregiver educational program improves quality of life and burden for cancer patients and their caregivers: A randomised clinical trial. *European Journal of Oncology Nursing*. 17(6): 870–876.

Bell, J.M. and Wright, L.M. (1994) The future of family nursing: interventions, interventions, interventions. *Japan Journal of Nursing Research*. 27(2–3): 4–15.

Department of Health (2008) *End of Life Care Strategy: Promoting High Quality Care for All Adults at the End of Life*. London: Department of Health.

Ewing, G., Brundle, C., Payne, S. and Grande, G. (2012) The carer support needs assessment tool (CSNAT) for use in palliative and end-of-life care at home: a validation study. *Journal of Pain and Symptom Management* 46(3): 395–405.

Glaser, B. and Strauss, A. (1965) *Awareness of Dying*. Chicago: Aldine.

Hanson, E. (2003) Supporting families of terminally ill persons In O'Connor, M. and Aranda, S. (eds) P*alliative Care Nursing: A Guide to Practice*. Melbourne: Ausmed. pp. 329–350.

Ingleton, C., Morgan, J., Hughes, P., Noble, B., Evans, A. and Clark, D. (2004) Carer satisfaction with end of life care in Powys, Wales: a cross sectional survey. *Health and Social Care in the Community*. 12(1): 43–52.

Lee, C.M. (2010) Families matter: psychology of the family and the family of psychology. *Canadian Psychology*. 51(1): 1–8.

Kissane, D. and Bloch, S. (2002) *Family Focussed Grief Therapy*. Oxford: Oxford University Press.

Kristjanson, L., Hudson, P. and Oldham, L. (2003) Working with families In O'Connor, M. and Aranda, S. (eds) *Palliative Care Nursing: A Guide to Practice*. Melbourne: Ausmed. pp. 271–283.

McIntyre, R. (2002) *Nursing Support for Dying Patients*. London: Whur.

McIntyre R, Lugton J. (2005) supporting the family and carers In Lugton, J. and McIntyre, R. (eds) *Palliative Care: The Nursing Role*. Edinburgh: Elsevier.

Munroe, B., Oliviere, D. (2009) Communicating with family carers in Hudson P, Payne S (Eds) Family carers in palliative care: a guide for health and social care professionals. Oxford. Oxford University Press.

National Institute for Clinical Excellence (2004) *Guidance on Cancer Services. Improving Supportive and Palliative Care for Adults with Cancer. The Manual*. London: National Institute for Clinical Excellence.

Panke, J.T. and Ferrell, B.R. (2005) Emotional problems in the family' In Doyle, D., Hanks, G., Cherny, N. and Calman, K. (ed) *Oxford Textbook of Palliative Medicine* 3rd edn. Oxford: Oxford University Press.

Saunders, C. (2006) *Cecily Saunders Selected Writings 1958–2004.* Oxford: Oxford University Press.

Smith, P.C. (2001) Who is a carer? experiences of family caregivers in palliative care in Payne, S. and Ellis-Hill, C. (eds) *Chronic and Terminal Illness*. Oxford: Oxford University Press.

Smith, P. and Skilbeck, J. (2008) Working with family care-givers in a palliative setting In Payne, S., Seymour, J. and Ingleton, C. (eds) *Palliative Care Nursing Principles and Evidence for Practice* 2nd en. Maidenhead: Open University Press.

WHO definitions of palliative care available at: http://www.who.int/cancer/palliative/definition/en/

Zaider, T. and Kissane, D. (2007) Resilient families In Monroe, B. and Oliviere, D. (eds) *Resilience in Palliative Care Achievement in Adversity.* Oxford: Oxford University Press.

12

Palliative care emergencies

Introduction

Palliative care emergencies are situations arising for patients with life-threatening illnesses that might lead to death or severe impairment of quality of life if left untreated. Patients may deteriorate suddenly because of their existing illness or as the result of new problems. Patient prognosis will determine the treatment plan, active intervention may be appropriate for patients with a fair life expectancy, whilst for those close to the end of their life palliation and support for the patient and family would be indicated. Most situations resulting in a palliative care emergency are related to advancing disease, few patients have hope of cure. For this reason treatment options and aims need to be explained clearly so that the patient understands the implications of their current situation and any proposed treatment. Patients and families must, if they wish, be provided with sufficient information about anticipated outcomes and risks involved to enable them to make an informed choice about future treatment. The patient must be at the centre of any treatment decision and effective communication with the patient, friends and family is paramount to a successful and appropriate treatment. Some of these conversations will be pre-empted if the patient has previously had the opportunity to express their wishes through advanced care planning. This chapter will focus on the three common conditions associated with palliative care emergencies.

Fundamentals of Palliative Care for Student Nurses, First Edition. Megan Rosser and Helen C. Walsh.

Companion website: www.wiley.com/go/rosser_walsh/fundamentals_of_palliative_care

Learning outcomes

By the end of this chapter you will be able to

- identify the three common causes of a palliative care emergency;
- describe the presenting features of each condition;
- discuss the medical management of these conditions;
- discuss the nursing care provided for patients experiencing a palliative care emergency.

Palliative care emergencies

The more common conditions which constitute a palliative care emergency are spinal cord compression, superior vena cava obstruction (SVCO) and hypercalcaemia (Rosser, 2007). These conditions are generally the consequence of advancing malignant disease but may occur in other patient groups. Many patients presenting with one of the conditions could survive for many months after the event, therefore initial presentation needs to be regarded as an emergency in order to reduce the chance of severe and permanent damage occurring. Early intervention is vital in order to maintain the patient's quality of life for as long as possible. It is, therefore, important that nurses are able to recognise the early signs of these conditions in order to liaise with members of the multiprofessional team to ensure prompt treatment.

Spinal cord compression

Spinal cord compression occurs when pressure is exerted on the spinal cord by bone, soft tissue, tumour or infection. There are a number of causes of cord compression; this section will focus on malignant spinal cord compression. Guidelines about diagnosis and management of malignant spinal cord compression should be developed by every cancer network (NICE, 2008) so nurses should be able to contact the local cancer centre for advice about management of a patient with suspected cord compression.

Causes of spinal cord compression

- malignancy – metastatic spread (commonest);
- trauma;
- prolapsed disc;
- osteoarthritis;
- rheumatoid Arthritis;
- orthopaedic conditions such as spondylosis, kyphosis.

(Acutemed, 2013).

Spinal cord compression occurs in 5–10% of all cancer patients and is most common in patients living with breast, lung or prostatic cancers (Downing, 2001). It is usually caused by metastatic spread to the vertebrae (Salt, 2003). If cord compression is not correctly diagnosed or not considered by the medics to be an emergency, treatment will not be instigated within the twenty four hour window suggested by NICE (2008), consequently permanent neurological damage can result. The aim of swift accurate diagnosis and treatment is to maintain or restore motor function in patients who otherwise face the rest of their life with diminished mobility, continence and independence. The principles underpinning the correct approach to a suspected cord compression are highlighted in Fact box 12.1:

Fact Box 12.1

- Rapid diagnosis and treatment of spinal cord compression is vital.
- The outcomes of treatment are related to patients' level of function at time of presentation.
- 70–80% of patients walking at presentation will continue to walk following treatment.
- Only 5–10% of patients unable to walk at presentation will regain that function.

(Cervantes and Chirivella, 2004).

Symptoms of spinal cord compressions

Patients who are described by themselves, or their carers as 'going off their legs' should set alarm bells ringing in the nurse's mind and a full neurological assessment must be requested from the GP or medical team.

Pain is the primary presenting symptom of spinal cord compression and may precede other symptoms by months, therefore patients with a history of cancer who present with back pain should always be presumed to have spinal cord compression until proven otherwise (Watson, 2006). Aspects of the pain experienced by patients with spinal cord compression are distinctly different from other types of back pain; it is generally described as a dull ache which does not respond to normal analgesics and is exacerbated by sneezing or coughing. The most distinctive feature is that pain is worse when lying down and relieved by standing (Cervantes and Chirivella, 2004). Other diagnostic signs and symptoms of spinal cord compression are listed in Table 12.1

Table 12.1 Signs and symptoms of spinal cord compression.

- pain – in back, chest or abdomen – depending on the level of the tumour;
  dull ache
  worse when lying down, increasing overnight
  exacerbated by coughing, sneezing
  relieved by standing
- tenderness at the site of tumour;
- motor weakness – weakness of legs, difficulty in standing/walking;
- sensory alterations – numbness, tingling;
- bladder and bowel sphincter dysfunction – incontinence, retention, constipation.

Assessment of spinal cord compression

Assessment for suspected cord compression includes

- accurate medical history;
- neurological and physical examinations;
- pain assessment and investigations;
- MRI scan.

Cervantes and Chirivella (2004), NICE (2008)

The management of spinal cord compression

The aim of any treatment for confirmed spinal cord compression is to preserve or restore neurological function. The key to successful treatment of spinal cord compression is speed, the earlier the treatment the more likely the recovery of function. This is exceptionally important because up to one third of patients presenting with spinal cord compression will live at least a year after the symptoms develop (Rajer and Kovac, 2008).

Radiotherapy and high dose steroids are generally the treatment of choice (Cervantes and Chirivella, 2004). Therefore as soon as suspicion of compression occurs there is the need to involve the oncologist immediately. A stat dose of dexamethasone 16 mg IV is likely to be prescribed with subsequent daily oral doses, reducing gradually after radiotherapy has been completed. Other medications which may be prescribed for patients with spinal cord compression will be analgesics according to the WHO analgesic ladder, likely to include non steroidal anti-inflammatory drugs (NSAIDs) for bone pain and possibly opioid analgesics. The nurse should advise the patient about possible side effects and observe for signs of adverse reactions. Chemotherapy may be prescribed for patients with chemosensitive tumours (Downing, 2001).

Spinal decompression surgery may be indicated if

- the compression is the first manifestation of malignancy;
- the tumour is not radiosensitive;
- the spine is unstable;
- the compression is caused by a single metastasis.

(Cervantes and Chirivella, 2004).

Nursing care for these patients will follow trust guidelines for patients following spinal surgery.

Activity 12.1

Think about the nursing care the patients with spinal cord compression will need.

Nursing care will be governed by an individual assessment of each patient and their level of independence but will include

- administration of prescribed medication and observation for side effects;
- skin care as per trust/Health board policy for patients receiving radiotherapy;

- bowel and bladder care;
- rehabilitation care in collaboration with therapists;
- education and support about changed situation/ level of dependency;
- pressure area care;
- care of personal hygiene;
- liaison with MD team to ensure timely and appropriate transfer of care once the patient is fit for discharge.

Superior vena cava obstruction (SVCO)

SVCO occurs when the superior vena cava is compressed or occluded and the circulatory flow is obstructed causing severe reduction in venous return from the head, neck and upper extremities. 90% of cases occur because of malignancy but the benign causes of SVCO, such as central venous catheters and cardiac devices are on the increase (Warner and Uberoi, 2013). SVCO occurs in 3–8% of patients with cancer (Downing 2001). 90% of cases of SVCO are caused by primary lung tumours, lymphomas and metastatic tumours, with almost 85% being caused by lung tumours (Cervantes and Chirivella, 2004).

Because of the venous obstruction and compression intravenous pressure increases and collateral circulation develops. In the vast majority of cases the development of SVCO is quite insidious and patients present with a variety of signs and symptoms as presented in Table 12.2. For most patients the symptoms are uncomfortable rather than life threatening so SVCO is not a 'true emergency', however, in the event of severe or rapid presentation of SVCO where there has been little time for collateral circulation to develop, symptoms may be immediately life threatening (Watson, 2006).

Table 12.2 Signs and symptoms of SVCO (Cervantes and Chirivella, 2004).

- Venous distension neck and chest
- Facial oedema
- Plethora – dilation of superficial blood vessels
- Proptosis
- Stridor
- Oedema of arms
- Neck and facial swelling (especially eyes)
- Cough
- Dyspnoea
- Pressure symptoms, head fullness/headache
- Hoarseness
- Nasal congestion/epistaxis
- Haemoptysis
- Dizziness
- Dysphagia
- Syncope

Symptoms may be exacerbated by bending forward or lying down

Assessment of SVCO

SVCO may be detected on a straight chest X-ray and confirmed by CT scan, histology needs to be confirmed if possible to ensure provision of the most appropriate treatment. Survival following SVCO generally depends on the underlying cause as opposed to the severity of symptoms although dysphagia, hoarseness and stridor are accepted to be poor prognostic factors. If SVCO is left untreated it will progress to produce altered mental state including stupor, coma, seizures and ultimately death (Watson, 2006).

The management of SVCO

The aim of care is to relieve symptoms and possibly cure the underlying disease. Treatment decisions will be determined by the histology of causative tumour and patient health and prognosis. Stenting is becoming the treatment of choice in many cancer centres and has higher success rates in the relief of symptoms than radio/chemotherapy (Rowell and Gleeson, 2001; Warner and Uberoi, 2013). Patients may also receive radiotherapy or chemotherapy depending on tumour histology and sensitivity. If prognosis is very short the focus of care is symptom control. The efficacy of steroids in SVCO is unproven (Rowell and Gleeson, 2001) and may be prescribed as a matter of personal preference of clinicians. Steroids may be the primary treatment choice if the patient is too ill for more aggressive treatment or the treatment plan is unclear (Salt, 2003).

Activity 12.2

Think about the nursing care that patients with SVCO will need.

Nursing care will include

- appropriate care for the breathless patient, if the patient is very breathless bed rest may be encouraged with the patient sitting well upright, supported by pillows, or in a comfortable chair if more comfortable;
- trial of oxygen – discontinue if no relief provided;
- psychological care for the patient, families and friends;
- support and education about condition and treatment;
- pressure area care;
- care of personal hygiene and elimination needs;
- care relevant to treatment modality – chemo or radiotherapy if ordered.

Hypercalcaemia

Hypercalcaemia is diagnosed when the corrected serum calcium level is above 2.6 mmol/L (Salt, 2003). The most common causes of hypercalcaemia are primary hyperparathyroidism and malignancy (Saini and Mesioye, 2010). Malignancy-related hypercalcaemia is the most common metabolic disorder associated with cancer and occurs in 10–20% of all cancer patients (Mount Vernon, 2011). Increased release of calcium from the bones is the main factor contributing to hypercalcaemia in cancer patients. Contrary to common belief, bone metastases are not always present. Twenty percent of patients with tumour-related hypercalcaemia do not have bone metastases, with hypercalcaemia occurring as a paraneoplastic phenomenon causing altered bone metabolism (Salt, 2003). The prevalence of hypercalcaemia is highest in patients with multiple myeloma, prostate and breast cancer, followed by patients with small cell lung cancer and lymphoma (Mount Vernon, 2011).

Common signs and symptoms are presented in Table 12.3; some of the symptoms may be confused with general symptoms of advancing disease. Nurses need to be mindful of the signs and symptoms so they are able to identify patients at risk of developing hypercalcaemia and respond accordingly.

Assessment of hypercalcaemia

Whilst a comprehensive nursing assessment will identify the presence of symptoms, hypercalcaemia is confirmed by a blood test to ascertain the corrected serum calcium level.

Management of hypercalcaemia

Control of hypercalcaemia will not ultimately affect prognosis but may improve the patient's symptoms and quality of life, treatment is indicated when serum levels are above 2.8 mmol/L (Salt, 2003). The aim of any intervention is to restore normal levels of serum calcium, thus relieving signs and symptoms. Tumour induced hypercalcaemia is associated with a low survival rate (Heatley, 2004) and patients tend to experience repeated episodes of hypercalcaemia.

Table 12.3 Signs and symptoms of hypercalcaemia.

• Fatigue • Malaise • Anorexia • Nausea • Vomiting • Confusion • Bone pain • Polydypsia, polyurea • Constipation • Weakness • Cardiac arrhythmias
Increased neurological symptoms if 3.5 mmol +: – Confusion – Sleepiness – Lethargy – Coma

Ultimately a patient may present with a final episode of hypercalcaemia where corrective treatment is no longer appropriate and end of life care becomes the focus.

Reduction of serum calcium levels is achieved by

- IV hydration with normal saline;
- IV bisphosphonates – for example, zoledronic acid, pamidronate;
- Steroids.

Bisphosphonates are a group of drugs which inhibit osteoclast activity. Osteoclasts are responsible for bone breakdown and resorption as part of maintaining bone homeostaisis. Degradation and resorption of bone is vital to bone remodelling and releases calcium into the circulation. Inhibition of osteoclast activity therefore reduces the level of circulating calcium, thus correcting episodes of hypercalcaemia. Maintenance therapy can be provided by continued administration of bisphophonates, either orally or by regular infusion as a day patient. Dosage and frequency of treatment will be determined by the rate of the increasing calcium levels.

Activity 12.3

Think about the nursing care that patients with hypercalcaemia will need.

Nursing care of patients with hypercalcaemia will include

- care of gastro-intestinal symptoms of constipation, nausea and vomiting;
- ensuring the safety of drowsy or confused patients;
- stringent mouth care;
- assistance with activities of daily living in accordance with patient capability to self care.

Depending on the initial response to treatment and the anticipated prognosis of the patient further cancer treatments may be offered. These decisions will be governed by factors such as histology, extent of disease, rate of progression, prognosis and patient choice. Patients and their families will need support if it is an episode of hypercalcaemia that presents as the likely terminal event.

Conclusion

Nurses spend a lot of time with their patients and may be either the first health care professional to recognise subtle changes in the patient's condition or the person to whom carers or patients voice their concerns. It is important that nurses are familiar with the signs and symptoms of the common palliative care emergencies. They need to be able to respond quickly and appropriately if they feel that the patient is developing one of the conditions that warrant rapid assessment and treatment in order to maintain the patients' quality of life and well being. Rapid communication with the doctors is vital to ensure the patient is referred immediately for the correct treatment. Other members of the multi-disciplinary team may become involved with the patient for rehabilitation following the acute episode.

Glossary

Bisphosphonate	Drug which inhibits osteoclast activity.
Cardiac arrhythmia	Irregular heart beat.
Chemotherapy	Use of drugs to kill off or control cancer cells.
Collateral circulation	Development of blood circulation through minor vessels that become enlarged and join adjacent vessels when a major vein or artery is impaired.
Dexamethasone	A corticosteroid used to treat inflammation and reduce swelling.
Dysphagia	Difficulty in swallowing.
Dyspnoea	The distressing awareness of the process of breathing.
Epistaxis	Nose bleed.
Haemoptysis	Coughing up blood.
Hypercalcaemia	Serum levels of calcium above 2.6 mmol/L. It causes a number of symptoms including nausea and vomiting and is ultimately fatal if left untreated.
Lethargy	Lacking in energy, feeling tired.
Non Steroidal Anti-inflammatory Drugs	Group of drugs with anti-inflammatory properties used to to treat inflammation, pain or fever.
Opioid analgesics	Synthetic drugs that bind to opioid receptors in the body to provide analgesic effect; include morphine, diamorphine, fentanyl, oxycodone.
Osteoclasts	Cells which mediate bone breakdown and resorption.
Palliative care emergency	Situations that arise for patients with life- threatening illnesses which if left untreated may lead to death or compromised quality of life.
Paraneoplastic	Changes that occur in tissues due to the presence of cancer elsewhere in the body, possibly arising from hormonal and immunological influences and responses.
Polydypsia	Experience of excessive thirst.
Polyurea	Passing excessive amounts of urine.
Prognosis	Anticipated length of time that a patient has to live.
Proptosis	Bulging eyes.
Radiotherapy	Controlled use of high energy X-rays to treat a variety of cancers.

Spinal cord compression	Compression of the spinal cord through pressure from bone, soft tissue, tumour or infection.
Steroids	(Corticosteroids) anti-inflammatory drugs prescribed for wide range of conditions.
Stridor	Loud, harsh, high pitched respiratory sound.
Stupor	Reduced level of consciousness and awareness.
Superior vena cava obstruction	Compression or occlusion of the superior vena cava, causing reduced venous return from the head and neck and upper extremities.
Syncope	Fainting.

Patient scenario

Mr George Smith is a 60-year-old man who was diagnosed with stage B cancer of the prostate two years ago. George underwent a course of radiotherapy shortly after diagnosis and now receives three monthly injections of Zoladex to control his disease. George lives with his wife Phyllis; they have been married 40 years and have two daughters who live away with their own families. George has been very well until recently. He has been to see the GP today, complaining of a persistent dull ache in his lower back, the pain is worse at night and he gets some relief when he stands up. He has also experienced some pins and needles in his legs and is finding it increasingly difficult to have his bowels open.

Being familiar with George's past medical history the GP suspects the possible diagnosis of malignant spinal cord compression. The GP contacts the oncology team at the local cancer centre who treated George and arrange for an urgent MRI. The MRI confirms spinal metastases and George is admitted for a five day course of radiotherapy and a course of high dose steroids (16 mg dexamethasone).

Activity 12.4

Describe the nursing care that you think would be appropriate for George. Compare your answers to those in the following text.

Information	at George's own pace, try and go with the doctor when they are speaking with George so you know what he has been told and can assess what he understands from the conversation. It may or may not be necessary to repeat or to supplement information.
Support	for George and Phyllis and their daughters regarding confirmed progression of his disease, Altered future and expectations.

Radiotherapy	skin care as per local policy, hygiene, assessment and protection. Remind George about possible side effects which might develop a couple of weeks after treatment, they should be milder than those he experienced during initial treatment and will include possible tiredness, skin soreness and gastro-intestinal symptoms depending on the field of treatment.
Steroids	given as one dose in the morning – to mimic the body's natural corticosteroid patterns, thus reducing risk of side effects. Observe for side effects (Chapter 5) and report.
Pain	administer analgesia as prescribed; will probably include NSAIDs and opioids. Review and report effect of analgesia. Observe for side effects (Chapter 5) and report. Help with positioning as necessary in order to promote comfort.
Activities	assist with daily living activities as required by George.
Elimination	monitor and record bowel and bladder function.
Immobility	prevention of potential complications, skin bundles, pressure area care, assess need for anti-embolus stockings. Encourage mobilising as allowed and as tolerated.

References

Acutemed (2013) *Spinal cord compression* Available at http://www.acutemed.co.uk/diseases/Spinal+Cord+Compression# [accessed 18 February 2014].

Cervantes, A. and Chirivella, I. (2004) Oncological emergencies. *Annals of Oncology.* 15(Supplement 4): iv299–iv306.

Downing, J. (2001) Acute events in cancer care In Corner, J., Bailey, C. (eds) *Cancer Nursing: Care in Context*. Oxford: Blackwell Science.

Heatley, S. (2004) Metastatic bone disease and tumour induced hypercalcaemia: treatment options. *International Journal of Palliative Nursing.* 10(1): 41–46.

Mount Vernon (2011) *Mount Vernon Cancer Network Guidelines for the Management of Hypercalcaemia in Malignancy*. Available at http://pro.mountvernoncancernetwork.nhs.uk/assets/Microsoft-Word-Management-of-Hypercalcaemia-in-Malignancy-guidelines-v1-2-May-4.pdf [accessed 18 February 2014].

National Institute for Health and Clinical Excellence (2008) *Metastatic Spinal Cord Compression: Diagnosis and Management of Adults at Risk of and with Metastatic Spinal Cord Compression*. London: NICE.

Rajer, M. and Kovac, V. (2008) Malignant spinal cord compression. *Radiology Oncology.* 42 (1): 23–31.

Rosser, M. (2007) Palliative care emergencies 1: diagnosis. *Nursing Times.* 103 (33): 28–29.

Rowell, N.P., Gleeson, F.V. (2001) *Steroids, radiotherapy, chemotherapy and stents for superior vena caval obstruction in carcinoma of the bronchus*. Cochrane Review. Cochrane Library.

Saini, B. and Mesioye, A. (2010) What is the diagnosis? Familial Hypocalcuric hypercalcaemia or primary hyperparathyroidism with vitamin D deficiency. *Journal of the American Medical Directors Association.* 14(3): B9–B10.

Salt, S. (2003) Tripwires in palliative care In Thomas, K. (ed) *Caring for the Dying at Home*. Oxford: Radcliffe.

Warner, P. and Uberoi, R. (2013) Superior vena cava stenting in the 21st century. *Post graduate medical journal on line.* 10.1136/postgradmedj-2012-131186.

Watson, A.C. (2006) Urgent syndromes at the end of life In Ferrell, B.R. and Coyle, N. (eds) *Textbook of Palliative Nursing*. 2nd edn. Oxford: Oxford University Press

13

Nursing care at end of life

Introduction

As patients approach the end of their lives, they become increasingly dependent on others to provide care and keep them as comfortable as possible. This is the nurse's domain and as observed by Virginia Henderson, many decades ago, is one area where nursing really comes into its own.

> The unique function of the nurse is to assist the individual, sick or well, in the performance of those activities contributing to health or its recovery (or peaceful death) that he would perform unaided if he had the necessary strength, will or knowledge.
>
> *Nursing Henderson, 2009*

For nurses (and other health care professionals) who see their role as helping promote health and recovery, palliative care and end of life care can be particularly challenging; for others the opportunity to care for someone towards and at the end of life can be extremely fulfilling, although difficult at times. This chapter focuses on care needed as patients approach the end of their life.

Fundamentals of Palliative Care for Student Nurses, First Edition. Megan Rosser and Helen C. Walsh.

Companion website: www.wiley.com/go/rosser_walsh/fundamentals_of_palliative_care

Learning outcomes

By the end of this chapter you will be able to

- identify when a patient is approaching death;
- discuss the nursing care of the dying patient;
- consider the nurse's role after death;
- recognise barriers to optimal end of life care.

Activity 13.1

If you have looked after someone who was dying, think about how you, or the staff nurse, knew the patient was dying?

Recognising that a patient is dying

To provide good nursing care for a dying patient it is important to be able to recognise when patients are approaching the final stage of their life. Common signs that you might notice in dying patients include:

- profound weakness
- gaunt appearance
- drowsiness
- disorientation
- diminished oral intake
- difficulty taking oral medications
- poor concentration
- skin colour changes
- temperature changes.

Faull and Nyatanga, 2005: p385.

When the patient is very close to death there may be a more rapid deterioration in the above signs. When patients are dying it is important that all unnecessary treatments are stopped to ensure that the burden on the patient is minimal. Review of medications is one of the central tenets of end of life care. Drugs that are providing symptom relief should be continued via the most appropriate route; this may be by continuous sub-cutaneous infusion via a syringe driver. Other drugs should be discontinued.

End of life care

Truly holistic care is vital when patients are dying and should be extended to include the patient's family and close friends, where possible. End of life care is the term that encapsulates all aspects of care required by dying people and their families. It includes continued management of pain and other symptoms and provision of psychological, social, spiritual and practical support, all of which have been discussed in previous chapters. From the 10 underpinning principles of end of life care (DH, 2008), the following are the most relevant at this point in the patient's journey:

- people to be treated with dignity and respect at the end of their lives;
- to ensure pain and suffering is minimised and optimal quality of life maintained;
- all people to have access to physical, psychological, social and spiritual care;
- services to be well coordinated to ensure seamless service;
- high quality care to be provided in the last days of life and following death in all settings;
- carers to be supported during a patient's illness and after their death.

Following the recommended phasing out of the LCP (Department of Health, 2013) individual end of life care plans must still ensure the following:

- communication with the patient's family remains central to care; the family should be told when the patient is dying, how that death might occur and given the opportunity to ask questions;
- the family, where possible, is involved in decisions and discussion about resuscitation, hydration and nutrition;
- medications are reviewed and altered to ensure optimal pain and symptom management, including the prescription of PRN drugs to enable management of potential symptoms or situations that can be anticipated;
- appropriate holistic care is planned, implemented and regularly evaluated and changed if necessary.

What makes a good death?

There have been studies that have sought to identify what need to be present in order for a death to be 'good'.

Activity 13.2

List all the things that you believe contribute to a good death. Compare your answer to the points highlighted in Figure 13.1.

Between the academic and the lay interpretation of a good death there are many points which are agreed on and can be seen in Figure 13.1.

Activity 13.3

What nursing care do you think is important for patients who are dying?

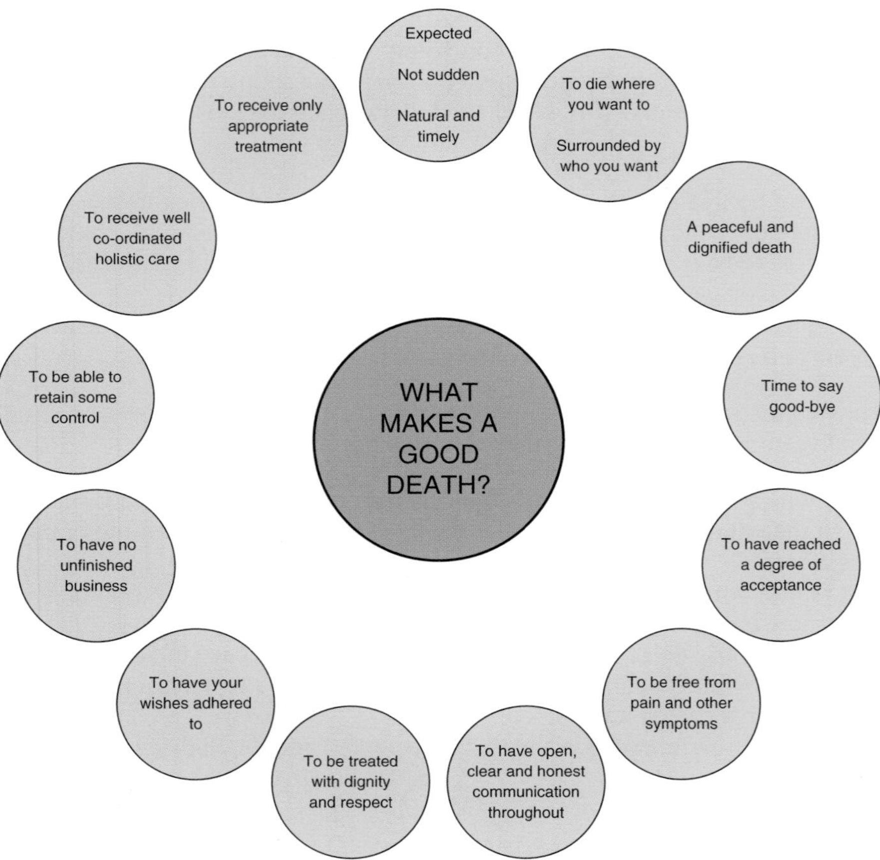

Figure 13.1 What makes a good death?

Physical nursing care for the dying patient

Good nursing care at this point will include close observation of your patient, both for the efficacy of pain or symptom management interventions and the gradual changes which herald the approach of death. While end of life care often includes supporting family and friends, the overall aim of all nursing care at the end of life is promotion of comfort for the patient. The nursing priorities for dying patients include

- mouth care;
- pressure area care;
- personal hygiene and elimination needs.

Mouth care

It has been said that the state of a patient's mouth is indicative of the level of nursing care received (Heals, 1993). Mouth care is a vital element of nursing care for all patients but is especially important for dying patients. Patients' mouths must be kept as clean and as comfortable as possible. Dying patients are particularly prone to dry mouths because of a number of factors including

- presence of oral thrush;
- drug side effects;
- mouth breathing;
- an inability to maintain their own mouth care regimes;
- reduced fluid intake.

Regular brushing with a soft toothbrush and toothpaste is the best way to keep the mouth fresh and moist if the patient can tolerate. An electric toothbrush may be easier for the patient to use and may enable him/her to retain independence longer. Dying patients can experience a number of oral problems.

- if the patient has oral thrush they need to be prescribed nystatin suspension. Dentures need to be soaked overnight either in a Milton solution or in nystatin suspension to eliminate the fungus.
- sore dry lips can be relieved by application of an unflavoured lip salve or KY jelly. (Vaseline is no longer used because it can dry lips further and also needs to be used with caution if the patient is using oxygen).
- a coated tongue can cause a great deal of distress and cause halitosis; some of the coating may be removed by the patient sucking 1/4 of an effervescent vitamin C tablet, or chewing part of a pineapple chunk if they are able to. (Neither of these interventions should be used long term because of the corrosive nature of citric acid).
- flavoured ice cubes can also help to maintain a moist oral mucosa.

Once the patient becomes too unwell to maintain their own mouth care it is imperative that you continue to carry out regular mouth care to prevent the patient experiencing discomfort, as long as it does not cause them distress. Patients may not tolerate a toothbrush; it can provoke a gagging reflex. Often it is sufficient to clean a dying patient's mouth gently with moistened mouth sponges. This may also be something that family members would like to do, so that they are able to continue to care for their relatives at the end of their life.

Pressure area care

Activity 13.4

How can you minimise the risk of dying patients developing pressure sore?

Dying patients are at high risk of developing pressure ulcers for a number of reasons. They are generally more underweight with more bony prominences, more malnourished and dehydrated than other patients and are less able to move around easily. They may also be incontinent. Pressure ulcers are painful and distressing so it is the nurse's duty to try and prevent them from developing and causing the patient more pain and discomfort. Patients' risk can be calculated using assessment tools such as the Braden scale (Bergstrom *et al.*, 1987), the Norton scale (Norton *et al.*, 1979) or the Waterlow scale (Waterlow, 1985).

Using the four key areas assessed in skin care bundles (1000 lives plus, 2013) as a guide enables you to identify the areas of concern and plan care accordingly.

1. **S**urface the patient is lying or sitting on – as death gets closer, the patient is most likely to be nursed in bed or in a comfortable chair (if very breathless or scared of going to bed because of association with dying). It is important that pressure relieving mattresses and cushions are used to protect the patient's pressure areas.
2. **K**eeping the patient moving – this is more challenging as the dying patient is likely to have limited mobility and may, in fact, be moribund and immobile. A degree of movement can be maintained by regular repositioning of the patient. If the patient obviously does not like being turned, it is kinder and just as effective to use pillows to support the patient's body in order to maintain a 30° tilt. Great care has to be taken when moving the patients to ensure that there are no unnecessary shearing or dragging forces exerted; these are uncomfortable for the patient and also increase the risk of pressure ulcer development.

3. **I**ncontinence – dying patients may be incontinent, either of urine or faeces or both. Close observation and stringent perineal hygiene are vital in order to prevent skin excoriation which is extremely painful, and pressure ulcer development.
4. **N**utrition – oral intake is likely to be extremely limited at the end of life and it is inappropriate to be pushing food or fluids at this point, so this is the area that you are least able to make changes in relation to pressure ulcer risk. If, however, you are vigilant in the first three areas, it is likely that patients will not develop pressure ulcers even if they are malnourished and dehydrated.

Despite the most conscientious nursing care some patients will develop pressure ulcers, especially if the patient requests not to be moved or turned. These ulcers will need to be dressed appropriately with the emphasis on patient comfort as opposed to healing, as time is short. It may be necessary to request advice from the tissue viability nurses about best management, taking into account the patient's prognosis.

Personal hygiene needs

Most dying patients are completely reliant on nurses, carers or family members to meet their personal hygiene needs, which are important in maintaining comfort. When you are caring for someone who is dying you will carry out all necessary care, this will include offering the patient a bed bath. The bed bath may be carried out using the traditional methods involving the wash bowl, warm water and flannels or the more recent approach of bed bath wipes – the latter being more efficient, acceptable to patients and nurses and also less likely to introduce infection to the patient (Massa, 2010). The most important thing to remember when washing a patient is that the patient's privacy and dignity must be maintained, and that a patient does not have to have a wash if they do not want one. Patient comfort is paramount and if a full bed bath is going to cause the patient too much distress just offer him/her a freshen-up.

In addition to offering a bed bath, it is important to brush the patient's hair, to shave a male patient and other personal touches such as applying make-up if you know that that their appearance is important to them, however ill they are.

Urinary and/faecal incontinence is quite common in dying patients, often because the weakness associated with end stage disease makes it impossible for the patient to access toilet facilities or to use a bed pan or urinary bottle with ease. If incontinence is not attended to, it can cause distress to patients and families. Practical solutions which can be used to overcome the problem and maintain patient dignity and comfort include

- regular and stringent cleansing of perineum;
- use of incontinence sheets and pads;
- penile sheaths;
- urinary catheters;
- continued bowel intervention, if necessary.

Bronchial secretions ('death rattle')

Noisy breathing, often referred to as the 'death rattle', occurs when the patient is no longer able to cough up or to swallow secretions which then accumulate in the mouth and throat. It is accepted as a sign that death is approaching (Twomey and Dowling, 2013). The noise comes from the air passing through the secretions in the airways. Whilst it does not generally trouble the patient, it can be very distressing for those sitting with the patient. Mouth care can help to clear the oral secretions and changing the patient's position may be enough to help clear the secretions. Suctioning is helpful for some patients, but it is not always tolerated by patients and may cause more distress for the family.

Whilst the evidence base is not particularly strong, there are medications that might be used to reduce the amount of secretions; these are listed in Table 13.1.

Terminal restlessness

One of the factors contributing to a good death for most people is the concept of a peaceful death. Whilst Dylan Thomas (1952) urged his father 'do not go gentle into that good night' most people hope that the person they love dies peacefully. As death approaches, about 10% of dying people do become restless (Salt, 2003) and this can be distressing for the patient, their friends and families and to the professionals who are committed to facilitating a peaceful death. Terminal restlessness occurs for a number of reasons and varies in the intensity of presentation.

Table 13.1 Drugs used to reduce bronchial secretions in terminal phase.

Drug	Route	Side effects
Glycopyrrolate	SC/IM/IV	Potent anti-secretory Less sedating May cause dry mouth, urinary retention
Buscopan	PO/SC/IM/IV	Not as sedating as hyoscine or scopolamine May cause tachycardia, dry mouth, retention of urine
Hyoscine hydrobromide	SC/IM/IV/ transdermal (scopoderm)	Can cause sedation, hallucination, agitation

Activity 13.5

Make a list of all the things you think might make someone restless as they are approaching death – compare your list with the list in Box 13.1.

Box 13.1 Causes of terminal restlessness

Patient is uncomfortable
Full bladder
Urinary retention
Impacted bowel
Inadequate pain or symptom control
Drug toxicity – opioids
Emotional upset
Fear, anxiety, unresolved issues
Altered biochemistry – hypercalcaemia, uraemia
Cerebral anoxia
Stimulation of busy care environment – activity and lighting.

Assessment

If your patient becomes restless, think about

- their position in bed;
- their previous psychological/emotional state;
- their pain and symptom management;
- their bowel and bladder status;
- any possible metabolic problems such as uraemia, hypoxia, hypercalcaemia;
- possible side effects of drugs.

Management

All interventions need to be considered in relation to the current level of patient distress, the potential distress that interventions will cause for the patient or family, and the expected length of time the patient has left to live. This is where the multi-disciplinary decision-making process is so valuable; families should also be included in the decision-making process wherever possible. Some of the following interventions might help your patient to settle more easily.

- help patients to get into a more comfortable position in bed or chair;
- facilitate unfinished business where possible – help people to say good byes;
- if your patient's bladder is full, it may be necessary to pass a urinary catheter; urinary retention may occur if anti-cholinergic drugs have been prescribed for management of excessive bronchial secretions.

- if your patient is constipated then bowel intervention may be required using suppositories or microlax enemas.
- check that patient analgesia and other prescribed drugs are being delivered via the correct route providing optimal pain and symptom management.
- medication regimes may need to be reviewed.
- request visit from appropriate religious leader to offer prayer, blessing, support and religious/cultural rites for the dying patient.

Medical management

It may be necessary to add new drugs to the patient's regime in order to relieve the restlessness and agitation. The anticipated effect of administering the drugs will vary from taking the edge off the patient's anxiety to rendering them unconscious, if they are really distressed and agitated. It is important that if the plan is to sedate the patient that sufficient doses are given, as incomplete sedation can make the patient even more distressed.

Patients (if well enough) and families should be fully informed of the plan and the consequences wherever possible and given the opportunity to say good bye before the patient is sedated. Some terminal agitation is transient and it may be possible to reverse sedation after a few days and review the patient's level of distress.

Drugs commonly used to relieve terminal agitation and restlessness include

- Midazolam
- Levemepromoazine
- Haloperidol.

Diamorphine should not be used to try and sedate patients. If you have a placement in a specialist palliative care unit, you might see phenobarbitone used to sedate a patient experiencing very severe terminal restlessness.

The syringe driver

As the patient approaches death, it is very unlikely that they will be able to continue taking their medication orally. Drugs are most likely to be delivered via a continual sub-cutaneous infusion using a syringe driver. Syringe drivers enable practitioners to administer a number of drugs via the same system and it is easier to maintain a steady state of therapeutic drugs. Drugs are generally renewed every 24 hours or sooner, if dosages are altered or new drugs added to the regime. Administration of drugs via the syringe driver will be informed and governed by the local syringe driver policy which must be adhered to.

Activity 13.6

Think of the drugs you have seen being delivered via a syringe driver, try and remember why they were prescribed, that is, what the patient's problems were.

Drugs commonly used in a syringe driver are presented in Table 13.2.

Table 13.2 Drugs commonly used in syringe drivers in end of life care.

Drug	Indication
Diamorphine	Pain and/breathlessness
Haloperidol Metoclopramide Cyclizine	Uncontrolled nausea and vomiting
Hyoscine butylbromide	Abdominal cramps
Midazolam	Anxiety/terminal restlessness
Levomepromazine	Nausea and vomiting, restlessness
Hyoscine hydrobromide Glycopyrronium	Excessive respiratory secretions

Most practitioners would advocate combining no more than three drugs in one driver. Up to date information about compatibility of drugs, diluents to be used, maximum doses and so on, can be found in the British National Formulary (BNF), if not covered in your local policy. You can also ask for advice from the specialist palliative care team.

Being with a dying patient

Patients dying at home will most often die with only their family and friends there. In hospital and nursing and residential homes it is likely that a nurse or carer will be in close attendance. The nursing role at the end of life is one of 'being' with the patient and the family as opposed to 'doing' very much active nursing.

For most patients and their families this is generally a sad but peaceful time; nurses are there to offer extra support and to provide care and advice should relatives become concerned. Most professionals feel that patients should not die alone; therefore, if there are no friends or family present, ideally a nurse should be allocated to sit with the patient as they approach death. Key nursing activities at this point will include:

- clear and open communication with the family, encouraging families to come and stay with the patient if they want to and respect their privacy. Equally, respect their choice if they prefer not to be with the patient when they are dying. The choice is personal and not for professionals to judge.
- if family or friends are present, pop in frequently to check that they are OK and that the patient remains settled.
- remember, it is strongly believed that hearing is the last sense to go; explain this to the family and encourage them to talk to the patient. If you are the person sitting with the

patient you can do the same. Do not be tempted to speak across the patient as though they are not there and do not allow your colleagues to do so either.
- maintain gentle physical touch if it does not disturb the patient so the patient knows he/she is not alone.
- arrange for religious leader to come if required to offer religious sacraments and fulfil requested liturgies.

As death approaches you will notice a change in the patient's breathing, this may occur hours or sometimes days before death. What you will see is that the patient's breathing pattern becomes more irregular, there may be episodes of deep rapid breaths followed by episodes of slow shallow breaths where the patient appears to stop breathing all together for a while. This is known as Cheyne Stokes respiration. Explain this to the family so they understand what is happening. You, or the family, may think that the patient has died, only to hear them draw breath again. The patient's hands and feet become mottled and cold; families may need support around this time, if they are sitting holding the patient's hand. Lips and finger beds also become mottled. Eventually breathing will cease and the heart will stop beating and the patient dies. Allow family to stay as long as they want so they have time to start saying good bye to the person that they love. Some family members may want to be involved in laying the person out with you.

Nurse's role after death

It is acknowledged that the nurse's role extends beyond the patient's death into the realm of providing care for the deceased person and for the family. What was until recently referred to as last offices is now known as 'care after death' (National end of life care programme, 2011). The most important aspect of care after death for nurses are as follows:

- honouring spiritual and cultural wishes of the deceased person and the family;
- preparing the body for transfer (and for viewing should the family wish);
- maintaining the privacy and dignity of the deceased person;
- returning patient's possessions to the family.

There are useful publications which clarify the religious and cultural needs of different patient groups around the time of death and afterwards. If you are caring for patients in hospital, your trust or health board is likely to have a guide about caring for patients of different faiths. A useful guide available to nurses in all care settings is Neuberger's (2004) book about caring for dying patients of different faith.

Advanced care planning can overcome many of the problems that confront nurses who care for someone with different beliefs from their own. Advanced care planning enables patients to express their wishes for care up to and after death, so nurses should be aware of what is required and what is acceptable to the patient and family. Should you be in any doubt about how to care for someone of a particular culture or faith as death approaches, ask the patient (if they can communicate) or a member of their family or faith group. Rather than offending them, the question is likely to make them feel acknowledged and respected.

Activity 13.7

Think about a time when you helped a member of staff care for a patient who had died – what did you do?

How did you find the experience?

Nursing care after death involves the laying out of the person; this is done partly to prepare the body for transport from the place of death to the funeral directors and also to prepare the person for the family to say good bye. The aim should be to make the patient look as nice as possible because this picture may stay in people's minds for a long time, if they look peaceful and pain free this can really help relatives in their bereavement.

Information about care after death can be found in local trust or health board policies, or the Royal Marsden Handbook. Laying someone out involves carrying out the personal care that you provided for them when they were alive. If the family were present at the death or have arrived since the patient died, it is good practice to ask them if they want to help lay the person out, some people will want to be included, others will not. You will probably find that the experienced nurses and health care support workers tend to talk to their patients when laying them out; students involved in laying out a patient for the first time often remark that the nurses treated the patient just the same as when they were alive, this is a good starting point as it suggests individualised dignified care at the end.

When laying someone out you will find that you will be expected to do the following:

- wash the patient;
- close their eyes (if they do not close damp gauze squares on the lids may help) and the mouth (use a pillow or a jaw support if it does not stay shut);
- brush their hair (into their normal style where possible);
- use pads to absorb any leakages (It is the responsibility of the mortuary staff to pack orifices if necessary, not the nurse);
- cap any IV lines and spigot catheters-these will be removed in the mortuary;
- check with family regards their wishes and if requested to – remove any jewellery in the presence of another member of staff and document and store jewellery accordingly. Tape any rings that have been left on the body and document that jewellery went with the patient;
- dress the patient – normally in a shroud unless the family has prepared specific clothes;
- place patient identity labels on patient as per local policy;
- wrap the patient in a sheet;
- place the patient in a body bag if there is any leakage;
- arrange for removal of the body or if at home advise the family to do so.

Most nurses feel that laying someone out is the last thing that you can do for your patient and is a privilege. As a student it can be quite a daunting and emotional task, especially if you have never seen a dead body before. The nursing standard has a website area for students to share their experiences of caring for dying patients which might be a useful source of support. With the support of a caring, sensitive mentor students will be able to use the experience positively to enhance learning and to say good bye to the patient.

Conclusion

End of life care involves the provision of sensitive, appropriate, good quality nursing care to patients and their families before and after the patient's death. Fundamental nursing skills are required in combination with knowledge about the dying process. Nursing dying patients may be informed and guided by national and local policies but is nothing without genuine compassion and care which promotes patient dignity, choice and comfort. Whilst caring for people who are dying is a privilege and very rewarding, it is not without cost to nurses and, therefore, it is very important that you heed the advice given in Chapter 15.

Glossary

Advanced care planning	Documented discussions between patients and professionals to enable patients to express their preferences for their care in the final months of life
Anti-cholinergic drugs	Drugs that block the action of the neurotransmitter acetylcholine in the brain
Bony prominence	Parts of bones that stick out, especially when patients have lost weight – for example, ankle joint, hip bones, vertebrae
Care after death	Previously referred to as last offices. Washing and 'laying out' the patient.
Cheyne stoke respiration	Abnormal breathing patterns with cycles of slow deep breaths and rapid shallow breaths generally seen in patients approaching death
Continuous sub-cutaneous infusion	Prescribed medications administered continually via the sub-cutaneous route using a syringe driver and giving set that ensures absorption of medication and maintenance of therapeutic dose
Death rattle	Lay term used by many to describe the noisy breathing arising from air passing over excess secretions in the patient's mouth and throat
End of life care	Care that helps all those with advanced, progressive and incurable illness to live as well as possible until they die
Halitosis	Bad breath
Hypoxia	Low levels of oxygen circulating in the blood

Hypercalcaemia	Serum levels of calcium above 2.6 mmol/L., which causes a number of symptoms including nausea and vomiting and is ultimately fatal if left untreated
Milton	Sterilising fluid which can be used to treat dentures infected with oral thrush (candida)
Nystatin	Anti-fungal suspension used to treat oral thrush (candida)
Oral mucosa	Moist lining of the mouth
Oral thrush	Yeast infection in the mouth, caused by a fungus called Candida albicans
Pressure ulcer	Breakdown of skin and underlying tissue because of interrupted blood supply as the result of prolonged pressure; the affected skin becomes starved of oxygen and nutrients and begins to break down, leading to an ulcer forming
Syringe driver	Small portable battery operated pump which administers continuous sub-cutaneous infusion of prescribed medications
Terminal restlessness	Distressing symptom that may occur in some patients at the end of life; patients can experience anguish, restlessness, agitation, confusion, delusions or hallucinations
30° tilt	Patient in bed lies at a 30° tilt, on one buttock with the sacrum tilted clear of the bed, patient supported by pillows to maintain position – allows relief of pressure on sacrum and spine
Unfinished business	Unresolved issues from the past that the patient wishes to resolve before their death, may include getting in touch with people, asking people for forgiveness, forgiving people
Uraemia	The presence of excess urea and other chemical waste products in the blood, caused by kidney failure in advanced disease
Urinary retention	Inability to empty the bladder completely

Patient scenario

Don Archer is a 65-year-old married man, who was diagnosed two years ago with end stage renal disease (ESRD) secondary to hypertension and ischaemic heart disease. Following an advanced care planning discussion about his treatment options and prognosis, Don made the decision to start haemodialysis with the option to review his treatment decisions with the team if he felt his quality of life was being compromised beyond a level acceptable to him.

Dialysis three times a week kept Don feeling quite well and enabled him to continue with some social activities and his favourite hobby of pottering in the garden.

Over the past two months Don's condition has deteriorated; he has become increasingly fatigued and breathless and he feels that his quality of life is becoming unacceptable to him. Don and his wife Lorna spoke with the renal consultant and renal nurse practitioner and a joint decision was made to stop haemodialysis. The next day the nurse practitioner met with Don and his wife again to check out what Don understood about the decision to stop dialysis and what his expectations about the future were. She also gave him the opportunity to review the end of life care he had initially stated he would like during the advanced care planning discussions at the time of his diagnosis. Following these discussions, it was agreed that Don would like to stay at home for as long as possible and to be admitted to his local community hospital for end of life care once Lorna could not cope. Don did not want to be a burden to Lorna and it was a joint decision that he should die in hospital.

Don wrote and signed an advanced statement confirming that he wanted palliative treatment only and that he wanted to die in the local community hospital. He also wrote an advanced directive stating that he did not want to be resuscitated.

Since Don stopped dialysis, the district nurse has been visiting daily to monitor Don's condition, to provide any necessary nursing care and to provide support to Lorna and Don. Following his visit today the district nurse has spoken to the GP reporting that Lorna can no longer care for Don at home and that they are requesting admission. The GP has arranged this with the ward.

On arrival at the ward, Don is very unwell; he and Lorna report that

he has become increasingly drowsy and is spending all his time in bed now;
he is no longer able to eat or drink;
he is becoming increasingly breathless;
he is experiencing persistent nausea with occasional vomiting;
his skin itches all over;
his legs are swollen.

Following assessment the GP decides to start Don on a syringe driver.

Activity 13.8

Which drugs would you expect to see in the syringe driver and why?

Syringe driver is likely to contain:

Haloperidol for nausea, which is most likely owing to uraemia, and
Diamorphine for breathlessness.

NB – the dosages of both drugs will be less than usual to prevent effects of toxicity because of Don's impaired renal function.

The syringe driver works well and Don settles; however, after 24 h he develops excessive respiratory secretions so the GP reviews his driver.

Activity 13.9

What drug do you think the GP might add to the driver to reduce Don's respiratory secretions?

Glycopyrronium

Again the dose will be less than usual because of impaired renal function.

Activity 13.10

What would your nursing priorities be for Don and Lorna?

Emotional support for Don and Lorna.

Observation of preferences stated in advanced statement and advanced directive – ensure that rest of the team are aware of their existence.

Attention to personal hygiene – check whether or not Lorna wants to help as she has been caring for Don up to this point.

Skin care – adherence to SKIN bundle and use of non-soap based cleansers (such as aqueous cream – which must be rinsed off) and emollients (such as E45) to try and relieve itch.

Pressure area care – regular turning if tolerated and use of pressure saving mattress.

Mouth care – regular cleansing with soft toothbrush and toothpaste as tolerated, gentle moistening with mouth sponges. Apply unflavoured lip salve or KY jelly to Don's lips to prevent them drying out.

Care of elimination and continence.

Support for Lorna throughout and after Don's death.

References

1000 lives plus (2013) *Making Pressure Ulcers a Thing of the Past*. Available at http://www.1000livesplus.wales.nhs.uk/news/20484 [accessed 22 February 2014].

Bergstrom, N., Braden, B.J., Laguzza, A., Holman, V. (1987) The Braden scale for predicting pressure sore risk. *Nursing Research*. 36(4): 205–210.

Department of Health (2008) *End of Life Care Strategy* Available at http://www.dh.gov.uk/prod_consum_dh/groups/dh_digitalassets/@dh/@en/documents/digitalasset/dh_086345.pdf [accessed 22 February 2014].

Department of Health (2013) *More Care, Less Pathway: A Review of the Liverpool Care Pathway* Available at https://www.gov.uk/government/uploads/system/uploads/attachment_data/file/212450/Liverpool_Care_Pathway.pdf [accessed 22 February 2014].

Faull, C., Nyatanga, B. (2005) Terminal care and dying in Faull, C., Carter, Y., Daniels, L. (eds) *Handbook of Palliative Care,* 2nd edn. Oxford: Blackwell Publishing.

Heals, D (1993) A key to well-being: oral hygiene in patients with advanced cancer. *Professional Nurse*, 8(6): 391–398.

Massa, J. (2010) Improving efficiency, reducing infection, and enhancing experience. *British Journal of Nursing.* 19(22): 1408–1414.

National End of Life Care Programme (2011) *Guidance for Staff Responsible for Care After Death.* Available at http://www.endoflifecare.nhs.uk/assets/downloads/Care_After_Death___guidance.pdf [accessed 22 February 2014].

Neuberger, J. (2004) *Caring for Dying People of Different Faiths* 3rd edn. Oxford: Radcliffe.

Norton, D., McLaren, R., Exton-Smith, A.N. (1979) *An Investigation of Geriatric Problems in Hospital.* 3rd edn. London: Churchill Livingstone.

Nursing Henderson (2009) Available at http://nursinghenderson2009.blogspot.co.uk/ [accessed 22 February 2014]

Nursing standard xxxx- http://nursingstandard.rcnpublishing.co.uk/students/dealing-with-your-first-death/carrying-out-last-offices [accessed 22 February 2014]

Salt, S. (2003) Tripwires in palliative care In Thomas, K. (ed) *Caring for the Dying at Home*. Oxford: Radcliffe.

Thomas, D. (1952) *The Poems of Dylan Thomas*, New York: New Directions.

Twomey S, Dowling M (2013) Management of death rattle at end of life. *British Journal of Nursing.* 22(2): 81–85.

Waterlow J (1985) A risk assessment card. *Nursing Times.* 27(49): 51–55.

14

Loss grief and bereavement

Introduction

This chapter introduces the theories of loss, grief and bereavement. While written in the context of palliative care, a lot of information presented in this chapter will be applicable to all clinical areas. There are central tenets which apply regardless of how someone dies, be it sudden and unexpected as a result of sudden illness, trauma or accident, or anticipated and expected as the final stage in a chronic illness. All those left to grieve will experience many similar responses to their loss; therefore, knowledge gained from this chapter will be applicable to any clinical placement. Your experience of observing grief following a death will vary depending on your clinical placement. In accident and emergency you may see relatives grieving following a sudden, unexpected death of a loved one, while in the community you may well be involved in supporting someone that you have visited for a while and have a relationship with (Walsh, 2008b). Loss and the associated feelings of grief are universal, as observed by Branter (cited by Haig, 1990):

> Only those who avoid love can avoid grief. The point is to learn from grief and remain vulnerable to love.

Fundamentals of Palliative Care for Student Nurses, First Edition. Megan Rosser and Helen C. Walsh.

Companion website: www.wiley.com/go/rosser_walsh/fundamentals_of_palliative_care

Learning outcomes

By the end of this chapter you should be able to

- identify normal responses to loss;
- consider the theoretical explanations of the bereavement experience;
- discuss the nurse's role in helping the bereaved.

Before reading more about loss, grief and bereavement, it is important to understand the key terms relating to loss.

- **Loss**: Being deprived of something/someone we value (Stroebe, 1992)
- **Grief**: The intense and painful pining for and pre-occupation with somebody or something, now lost, to whom or which one was attached (Parkes, 2007)
- **Bereavement**: An essential component of grief – to be robbed/deprived, to have something taken away, generally associated with loss through death (Thompson, 2012)
- **Mourning**: Outward expression of grief including rituals and actions performed in response to bereavement – often influenced by societal or cultural expectations.

To bring all these together:

> Bereavement is an event; grief is the emotional process; mourning the cultural process.
>
> *Oliviere et al., 1998: p. 121*

Coping With Loss

Activity 14.1

Think about the losses your patients have already faced and the losses they may face in the future.

Compare your answers with the list in Box 14.1.

Box 14.1 Losses that patients may experience

Health	Faculties	Independence
Self concept	Hearing	Mobility
Sight	Dignity	Role
Spouse	Security	Hope

(*continued*)

Box 14.1 Losses that patients may experience (*continued*)

Family	Communication	Faith
Friends	Safety	Future
Home	Companionship	Job
Positive body image	Finances	

As you can see, patients will experience a number of losses as the consequence of living with a life-limiting disease. Nurses are often involved in supporting patients experiencing loss, and it is good to remember that people respond to loss in a variety of ways.

Activity 14.2

Think about something or someone you have lost.

What kind of feelings, thoughts and behaviour do you recall experiencing?

Compare your thoughts with the list in Table 14.1.

Table 14.1 Responses to loss.

Emotional responses	Physical responses	Cognitive responses	Behavioural responses
Sadness Depression Anxiety Anger Guilt – self-blame Loneliness Fatigue Helplessness Shock Yearning Emancipation Relief Numbness	Hollowness in stomach Tightness in the chest Tightness in the throat Noise sensitive Sense of depersonalisation Breathlessness Muscle weakness Lack of energy Dry mouth	Disbelief Confusion Pre-occupation Sense of presence Auditory or visual hallucinations Lack of concentration and attention Memory loss Helplessness/ hopelessness Sense of distance/ detachment	Sleep disturbances Dreams of the deceased Appetite disturbances Absent-minded behaviour Irritability – expression of emotions Restlessness Searching, calling out Crying Social withdrawal, isolation Avoiding reminders of the deceased Visiting places/carrying objects that are reminders of the deceased Sighing Restless hyperactivity Treasuring objects that belonged to the deceased

From Worden (2010).

Common emotional responses to loss

Anger

Anger is a normal and natural response for patients facing death and for people experiencing the death of someone they love. It can hide underlying fears and eventually, if unresolved, may result in the angry person becoming isolated from others who could otherwise support them. Anger needs to be acknowledged but not fuelled. Anger can be directed at anyone and can be misplaced at times. The bereaved may be very angry with the person who is dying, or has died, for leaving them but find it hard to express that anger so it becomes directed at others. Patients may be very angry about having their life cut short, about the current and future impact of the disease, the perceived unfairness for some. It is important to try and ascertain the cause of the person's anger and explore that sensitively with them.

Activity 14.3

Think of all the things that could make a dying patient angry.

Depression

While some people experience what might be accepted as appropriate sadness when their life is coming to an end or when someone they love is dying or has died, some people will experience a period of reactive depression. These people demonstrate a sense of hopelessness, loss of self-esteem, feelings of guilt and in extreme cases express a wish to end their own lives. Proper assessment using depression screening tools and psychological support is indicated for these people – as a nurse you might be the one who initially picks up on the person's feelings and brings that to the attention of someone appropriate, be that the home manager, the GP, the ward manager or the social worker. You may still be someone that the person likes to talk to and you can support them by sitting with them and listening, working in collaboration with more experienced practitioners.

Anxiety

There may be numerous sources of anxiety for patients and their families including

- loss of the future
- pain
- symptoms
- dyspnoea
- loss of dignity/control
- treatments
- outcomes of treatment
- dying.

Anxieties can be reduced by establishing therapeutic relationships in which the patient and family have trust and confidence, listening to fears and giving genuine reassurance once the root of the anxiety has been identified. Do not give false hope because this will undermine the therapeutic relationship.

Denial

Denial is a common defence against grief and can be used consciously or subconsciously to soften the blow of loss. Most people who are bereaved will experience a period of denial until the truth of death and separation actually sinks in; this can take different lengths of time for different people. Some patients experience denial in response to their diagnosis and/or prognosis. Few patients maintain their denial as their disease progresses; failure of denial as a coping mechanism often manifests as anxiety. These patients need kind and sensitive support while they mobilise other more effective coping mechanisms. It is important to be honest with these patients, at the same time giving them some source of realistic hope.

Bereavement theories

As noted by Cobb (2004), nurses are well placed to offer early bereavement support and understanding because many people begin their bereavement in the company of nurses. It is, therefore, important for you to have some understanding of the processes involved in bereavement and the experiences of the bereaved.

For most bereaved people grief is a normal reaction that they are able to manage themselves with the support of good family and friends. There has been a tendency of some theorists to medicalise grief and to suggest necessary therapeutic interventions. For those experiencing 'straightforward grief' this is not the case, their experiences are a normal part of life. Those who 'get stuck' in their grieving may require psychiatric or psychological intervention. An understanding of the theories and models of bereavement will help to identify who is progressing through their grieving 'normally' and who might be in need of support.

Bereavement theories and models have evolved over time and it is true to say that 'grief is much more complex than any one model can allow' (Walter, 1997). Some of the earlier theories suggested that the bereaved progressed through a series of phases or stages in a linear fashion, implying that grief was an illness and that bereaved people were only healthy once they had progressed through all the stages. This encouraged the medicalisation of grieving as opposed to acknowledgment of the experience as a normal process.

Phases and stages

Elisabeth Kubler-Ross published a seminal piece of work in 1969 entitled 'On Death and Dying'. While working with people facing death (as opposed to people who had been bereaved), Kubler-Ross suggested that in reaction to a cancer diagnosis people went through five distinct stages:

- denial – it cannot be true, you have made a mistake;
- anger;
- bargaining – often with a higher power – if I give up …, if I behave better then please let me live longer;
- depression;
- acceptance – coming to terms with actual and anticipated losses.

The model was accepted by some as the definitive model of bereavement; its influence was widespread. Where the model was accepted, people were often expected to progress through all stages without deviation. More recently there have been criticisms in relation to the prescriptive, linear model and also the lack of a compelling evidence base. Regardless of the academic worth, Kubler-Ross is acknowledged for bringing the subject of death and dying into professional and public arenas and her work still contributes to patient care today. Whatever the criticisms, it remains true that people will experience some of these emotions during their bereavement.

Bowlby and Parkes (1970) built on Bowlby's earlier attachment theory to propose a four phase model of grieving. While both authors independently continued to refine this model, the basic phases remain unaltered and are as follows:

- **Phase one: numbness and shock** – this occurs immediately after the loss and the bereaved are numb, the death seems unbelievable, there is an element of denial. This is the body's natural defence mechanisms, which enable the bereaved to survive emotionally.
- **Phase two: yearning and protest** – this is a period of intense yearning which may last for months and involves the experience of varied emotions underpinned by the longing for the dead person to return. Emotions include crying, anger, anxiety and confusion.
- **Phase three: despair and disorganisation** – the bereaved person begins to withdraw and disengage from friends and activities and experiences periods of despair, disinterest and apathy.
- **Phase four: re-organisation** – the bereaved person starts to regain interest in life, finds renewed energy and inclination towards enjoyment. Life starts to become a little more normal and the bereaved person starts to make a new life without the dead person.

Tasks of mourning

The stages and the phases models suggest that the bereaved just pass passively through the stages. William Worden introduced the 'tasks of mourning', suggesting that the bereaved needed to take an active part in their grieving and recovery. Worden first introduced his theory in 1982 and has refined it over the years, with the most recent model being proposed in 2010. There are some similarities with the work of Bowlby and Parkes and the tasks identified are as follows:

- **Task one – to accept the reality of the loss** – accepting the reality that the person has died and is not coming back. Needs to happen at an intellectual and emotional level.
- **Task two – to work through the pain of grief** – feeling and expressing the grief. The pain should not be denied or avoided.
- **Task three – to adjust to a world without the deceased** – adjusting to life without the deceased at (a) a functional level, taking on roles of the deceased; (b) an internal level, adjusting your own sense of self, for example, being on your own instead of part of a couple; (c) at a spiritual level – how does the death impact upon the bereaved sense of beliefs, values and meaning, trying to make sense of it all.
- **Task four – to find an enduring connection with the deceased in the midst of embarking on a new life** – the bereaved establishes an enduring connection with the dead person that enables him/her to feel connected and also to get on with life. It is about finding an appropriate place for the dead person in their emotional life, a sense of connection.

(Worden, 2010)

Sociological models

All these models are widely used in health care but are considered by some to be rigid and prescriptive, giving rise to medicalisation of grieving through the perceptions of letting go and moving on. If the bereaved fail to pass/work through the stages, phases or tasks of grief, they are considered to be stuck in their grief and in need of interventions (Walsh, 2008a). However, it has to be acknowledged that all of these models provide insight into the grief experience and in fact Worden's latest model (2010) has addressed some of these criticisms with increased emphasis on relationships and the acknowledgement of continuing bonds in stage four.

More recent modules have tended to move away from the psychological and physical manifestations of grief to emphasise the social aspects of death. Modern theorists support the increasingly popular view that grief is ongoing, irresolvable but liveable through continuing bonds. Walter (1996) suggests from personal experience of significant bereavements that the purpose of grief is to construct a biography of the dead person, enabling the bereaved to assimilate memories of the dead into their ongoing lives, thus maintain a sense of connection. This biography is constructed through talking about the dead person with others who knew that person; the emerging narrative helps the bereaved to make sense of their lives in relation to their bereavement (Thompson, 2012). It is important to recognise shared memories, treasure possessions and talk about the deceased (Walsh, 2008b).

This sense of connection was formally proposed by advocates of the 'continuing bonds' theory (Klass *et al.*, 1996) who suggest that

- it is normal for the bereaved to maintain a connection with the deceased which is not static;
- the bereaved construct an inner representation of the deceased; the relationship diminishes but does not disappear;
- the emphasis is on negotiating and re-negotiating the measure of the loss over time;
- accommodation occurs rather than recovery, closure or resolution, that is, continual activity of seeking the meaning of the place deceased holds in the survivor's life and sense of self.

Establishing continuing bonds is constructive if it enables the bereaved to enjoy and use memories as part of their ongoing lives. It can become problematic if it becomes the raison d'être and gives rise to a sense of duty to maintain grieving at the cost of everything else. Ultimately, in a healthy bereavement the bereaved find ways through their sorrow to a relationship with their grief (and the deceased) that is liveable, having found a way to move on while also remaining in the past, reviewing memories and history at the same time as learning how to live (Moules *et al.*, 2004).

Dual process model

Finally, Stroebe and Schut (1999) introduced their theory of dual process of grieving which is a psychological approach to grief that recognises the social context of bereavement and acknowledges the need to cope with the loss itself as well as the resulting changes in life through the processes of mourning and adaptation. These two activities give rise to the concept of two orientations of bereavement – loss orientation and restoration orientation. Activities associated with either orientation are presented in Table 14.2.

The bereaved oscillate between the two states and as they emerge from their bereavement they spend more and more time undertaking restoration associated activities, spending less

Table 14.2 Activities associated with the dual process model.

Loss orientated	Restoration orientated
Grief work Intrusion of grief Letting go/continuing–relocating bonds/ties Denial/avoidance of restoration changes	Attending to life changes Doing new things Distraction from grief Denial/avoidance of grief New roles/identities/relationships

From Stroebe and Schut (1999).

time focussing on the loss and the associated emotions. This model allows many patterns of 'normal' grief and acknowledges the need to mourn and to adapt. It is suggested that there are differences in the readiness of men and women to adopt either orientation, women have been observed to spend more time in the loss orientated activities while men more readily immerse themselves in restoration activities.

Activity 14.4

Think about someone you know who has been bereaved – how can one of the bereavement theories help to explain their experience?

How do you think understanding some of the bereavement theories will help your practice?

Some people find bereavement more difficult to cope with and there are a number of risk factors associated with poor outcomes of grief; these risk factors have been identified by Parkes (1998) and presented recently by Worden (2010) as mediators of mourning. The factors are highlighted and explained in Table 14.3.

Helping the bereaved

Activity 14.5

Think about the bereaved you have cared for when you have been in placement. What expressions of grief have you observed?

Think about how you have seen the staff respond to those who are grieving.

What do you think were helpful interactions and why?

What do you think were less helpful interactions and why?

Table 14.3 Factors influencing the impact and outcomes of bereavement.

Factor	Explanation
Who the person was	Different impact with different relationships Spouse, child, friend, grandparent
Nature of the attachment/relationship	Strength of the attachment – intensity of grief matches intensity of love Security of the attachment – can the survivor survive without the other, level of dependency Ambivalence – those grieving the loss of someone they are ambivalent about often experience more problems in bereavement Conflict – history of conflict over years of the relationship or immediately prior to death may give rise to complication in bereavement
Nature of the death	Untimely death more difficult to grieve Bereavement following suicide is a unique and challenging experience Violent or traumatic deaths are difficult to deal with Multiple losses can cause 'bereavement overload' Stigmatised death – less social support available
Previous experiences	How have people dealt with previous losses? – resolved/continuing problems
Personality factors	Gender – men and women grieve differently and respond to different interventions Coping styles – healthy or unhealthy – problem solving, emotional coping, avoidance tactics Attachment styles – secure/insecure. Secure grieve and able to move on, insecure – complicated grieving Cognitive styles – tendency to optimism/pessimism Sense of self esteem and self efficacy – stronger better outcomes
Social variables	Level of support from family, friends and society and processes of communication. Better support and open communication results in better outcomes
Concurrent stresses	Experiencing high levels of disruption prior to or following death affects outcomes of grief negatively

From Parkes (1998), Worden (2010).

Bereavement is hard, not only for those who have been bereaved but also for those working alongside them. As observed by Bowlby (1980), 'The loss of a loved person is one of the most intensely painful experiences any human being can suffer, and not only is it painful to experience, but also painful to witness, if only because we're so impotent to help'. Nurses often say that they do not know what to do or to say when caring for the bereaved and some will actively avoid the bereaved if possible. Nurses are often present at a patient's death and offer immediate support to friends and families. While nurses are not often involved in providing ongoing bereavement support, it is useful to know what can help people during their bereavement.

The impact of losing someone you love is enormous and life changing as suggested by Hicks (2007).

> To watch someone you love leave you and the world you know is the most difficult thing to face. It is the very notion of being absolutely powerless to change the outcome. There is absolutely nothing else you can do but cry. You cry for all the life they will never see, and for yourself because you are left, left behind to carry on without them, to continue with life in a world without them in it. It seems impossible.

Most people survive their bereavement with the support of good friends and families, learning to live without the person who has died, learning to continue with a very different life and to review their view of the world, their expectations and their future. This is described by Parkes (2000) as the psychosocial transitions, which occur as the bereaved make the necessary adjustments to enable them to continue to live and to function.

Compassionate nurses want to care for the bereaved offering consolation, but experience the same concerns as lay people and are often worried about making the situation worse. How nurses interact with the bereaved is in part influenced by their personal experience, their beliefs and their values; therefore, nurses need to be self aware in order to provide sensitive support to the bereaved. It is also important that nurses look after themselves.

There are certain principles that are good to keep in mind when you are caring for people who have been bereaved. These principles include the following:

- everyone is individual;
- grief is individual;
- there are many influences on expression of loss/grief;
- there is no 'proper' way to grieve;
- it is good to encourage expression of grief;
- it is important to listen and validate people's thoughts and emotions, listen to what they are saying and be accepting of feelings and behaviour;
- it is important to be there for people who are experiencing loss;
- do not expect the bereaved to forget the past and start again;
- always remember - that patient could be you or someone important to you;
- look after yourself and your colleagues.

Activity 14.6

What help/information do you think people need in bereavement?

Most bereaved people who have the support of good friends and family will not require professional input such as bereavement counselling. It has long been acknowledged that

> the most positive factor in favour of a 'good' bereavement outcome is the presence of supportive friends or family who will allow the bereaved person to express their grief when, how and for as long as they want to.
>
> *Parkes, 1981*

People who are grieving require comfort, emotional and practical help from people who accept and understand their reactions. All bereavement support aims to facilitate the grief process, helping people to cope, thus preventing chronic or complex grief reactions. Bereavement support may be provided at the time of death, or immediately following, or may form part of an aspect of continuing care. NICE (2004) identifies a 3-component model of bereavement support:

Component 1 – people require information about experience of grief and how to access services.
Component 2 – some people require more formal opportunity to review and reflect befriending, self-help.

Component 3 – minority will require specialist input – psychological support or bereavement services.

Nurses are most likely to be involved at the time of death or very soon after, fulfilling the first component of the bereavement support model. Nurses are often in the situation of providing initial comfort following the death and giving information such as who to contact or what to do next, when to return to the hospital or care home to pick up the patients property and death certificate. Some nurses, particularly those working in the community, have the opportunity to visit families a day or so after the patient has died. This time is for offering condolences and also for checking out how the friends and family seem to be coping in the early days. If the district nurse is concerned then the GP can be informed.

There are some relatively simple but very effective ways in which nurses can help the bereaved even in the very early stages of their bereavement

- being there;
- being non-judgemental;
- listening to the bereaved's story;
- demonstrate some understanding;
- encourage them to talk about the deceased;
- tolerate silence;
- be familiar with own feelings about grief;
- offer appropriate reassurance;
- do not take anger personally;
- recognising your feelings may reflect what they are feeling;
- accept you cannot make them feel better;
- respect people's need not to talk;
- attend to your own needs.

In addition to being comfortable offering support in the immediate and acute stages of grief, it is important to be able to recognise those who are struggling with their grief and need referring on for more formal support such as a bereavement group or a befriending service or for professional help. Knowledge of the mediators of grief and the expected grief responses can help nurses to identify those who are not grieving well. Many people who join bereavement groups like being able to take advantage of the opportunity to meet with others in similar situations in order to share experiences and to give and receive support. People have found that being part of a bereavement group helped them by being listened to and understood; they found sharing information was helpful. They valued the opportunity to share with people outside of their normal social network and felt that members of the group cared for each other and looked out for each other (Firth, 2005).

Resolution of mourning

Theorists would have different outcomes that indicate the end of mourning; for Bowlby and Parkes, it would be at completion of the fourth phase, Worden would argue that it is on completion of the fourth task. Walter and Klass would suggest that it is a continued process, facilitated through continuing bonds.

Whatever the theoretical background, it is accepted that the acute mourning phase is complete when people are no longer consumed by grief and can think of the deceased person without pain. Pain is different from sadness; people will continue to experience sadness when they think about the deceased, this becomes less intense over time and happens less often. People feel re-invigorated, they spend less time grieving and are ready to join in with life again, adapting to their new role. Life will never be the same again but it can be worth living once more. People find memories comforting rather than painful. Although people will reach that point at different times, there is a widely accepted agreement that it takes around two years to recover from a significant bereavement if grief is unimpeded.

Conclusion

Nurses spend a lot of time caring for people who are facing various losses. The experiences of those facing loss are varied and their needs differ accordingly. When working with patients, nurses may find themselves supporting people facing the ultimate loss, life itself, and may be involved in some deeply searching conversations. The role of the nurse here is often one of listening, paraphrasing and reflecting as people strive to make sense of their changed situation and their future.

When caring for the bereaved, nurses tend to be involved in the early stages of grieving following the death of a patient. At this point nurses are again engaged as listeners as the newly bereaved tell their stories. The nurse is also involved in providing practical information and assessing how the bereaved may cope, deciding whether professional help might be necessary to support them in their grieving. However, for most people the support of close friends and family is all they need to help them get through their grief to a point where they are ready to engage with life again, albeit as a slightly different person.

Glossary

Bargaining	Third stage of Elizabeth Kubler-Ross's model of grief. Involves negotiation with some real or abstract higher power, asking for more time/less pain, and so on, in exchange for altered behaviour. It can be seen as an attempt to postpone the inevitable.
Befriending service	support for bereaved people from trained volunteers who have often experienced bereavement themselves. Provide practical advice and emotional support.
Bereavement	To be robbed/deprived, to have something taken away. Generally associated with loss through death.
Bereavement group	Group providing mutual support for people who have all experienced loss. May be led by recognised facilitator or by group members themselves.
Continuing bonds theory	Based on the belief that people maintain a relationship with the deceased and that this relationship is OK and healthy. The bereaved have a dynamic, continuing relationship with the deceased finding a changed but present place for the relationship.
Denial	Recognised defence mechanism which protects people from enormity of news. Refusal/inability to admit that something is happening or has happened, for example, life-threatening diagnosis or death.
Grief	The intense and painful pining for and pre-occupation with somebody or something, now lost, to whom or which one was attached.
Loss	Being deprived of something/someone we value.
Loss orientated activities	One of the two activities in Stroebe and Schuts dual process model of grieving. Activities which focus on aspects of the loss experienced include grief work, intrusion of grief and denial or avoidance of restoration activities.
Mediators of mourning	Factors which influence how people respond to bereavement.
Mourning	Outward expression of grief including rituals and actions performed in response to bereavement – often influenced by societal or cultural expectations.

Restoration orientated activities	One of the two activities in Stroebe and Schuts dual process model of grieving. Activities which focus on trying to adapt to the challenges arising from the loss experienced, includes attending to changes, doing new things, developing new roles and identity.
Yearning	Intense or overpowering longing (for the person who has died).

Patient scenario

You have been on placement in a nursing home for the past 6 weeks. During that time you cared for Amita an 89-year-old lady who was in the end stages of dementia. You became very fond of her because she reminded you of your great Nan who died from dementia last year.

Amita had been living in the nursing home for the past three years as it had become unsafe for her to stay at home. Her husband, Rahul, had been very reluctant to let Amita go into the home but had eventually realised he could no longer care for her. Amita settled into the nursing home and appeared to be happy there. Rahul visited every day trying to come at lunch time so he could help feed Amita; he would then spend the afternoon sitting with her, reading to her and listening to their favourite music together. They had been married for 68 years and had no children. They did have a good network of friends through the local bowls club and the local Indian society and temple.

During your fourth week Amita died peacefully with Rahul and you present. You were able to attend Amita's funeral in order to say good bye to her and also to represent the nursing home. Today Rahul has come to visit the staff to say thank you, you spend some time with him.

Activity 14.7

How would you expect Rahul to be?

What would your concerns be for Rahul in the future?

What would you do during the time you got to spend with Rahul?

Answer these and compare your answers to the comments below.

Question 1

Rahul is obviously in the very early stages of his bereavement and he still may not believe that Amita has died.

The funeral may have made this a little more of a reality as he has had to say good bye to her. That reality may make him very sad and he may or may not feel comfortable showing his emotions in front of you.

Rahul may say that he sees, hears or feels Amita around him.

Rahul may not be taking care of himself and may appear less well kempt than usual.

Rahul may have problems sleeping.

Rahul may feel that life is pointless without Amita to care for, to visit and to talk to. His role as husband has gone.

Question 2

Concerns for Rahul in the future would include the following:

What will he do with all the time he has on his hands, having spent every day with Amita for the past three years at least?

Will he make contact with his previous friends and support networks or will he become isolated in his grief?

Will he be able to find new purpose in life now his main role has gone?

Will he want to carry on living or will he welcome death as a release?

Will he look after himself or neglect himself?

Question 3

The most important thing is to demonstrate your willingness to just 'be with' Rahul and to take your cues from him.

Time would be best spent listening to Rahul telling his story if he wants to talk about Amita. Encourage him to talk about her, their life together before she became ill as well as their life since her illness.

Use your interpersonal skills to help Rahul express how he is feeling. Respect his emotions and do not try to make it all better, acknowledge that it will take time for Rahul to feel differently.

Once you have given Rahul the option to share his feelings respect that he may not want to talk, and do not force the issue.

Keep the silences, allow Rahul time to gather his thoughts and emotions if he is finding it difficult to talk about things.

Share your thoughts and feeling about Amita – it helps relatively to know that their loved one was important to other people too. Be aware of your own emotions and needs around Amita's death – talk to someone at the nursing home afterwards if you found being with Rahul upsetting.

References

Bowlby, J., Parkes, C.M. (1970) Separation and loss within the family in Anthony, E.J. (ed) *The Child in His Family* New York: Wiley. pp. 197–216.

Bowlby, J. (1980) *Attachment and Loss* Volume 3. *Loss, Sadness and Depression*. New York: Basic Books.

Cobb, M. (2004) Care and support of bereaved people in Payne, S., Seymour, J., Ingleton C. (Eds) *Palliative Care Nursing: Principles and Evidence for Practice*. Maidenhead: Open university Press pp. 490–501.

Firth, P. (2005) Groupwork in palliative care In Firth, P., Luff, G, Oliviere, D. (eds) *Loss, Change and Bereavement in Palliative Care*. Maidenhead: Open University Press.

Haig, R.A. (1990). *The Anatomy of Grief: Biopsychosocial and Therapeutic Perspectives*. Springfield, IL: Charles C Thomas.

Hicks, G. (2007) *One Unknown* London: Rodale.

Klass, D., Silverman, P.R., Nickman, S.L. (1996) *Continuing Bonds New Understanding of Grief*. Philadelphia: Taylor & Francis.

Kubler-Ross, E. (1969) *On death & dying* London: Tavistock.

Moules, N.J., Simonson, K, Prins, M, Angus, P, Bell, J.M. (2004) Making room for grief: walking backwards and living forwards. *Nursing Inquiry* 11(2): 99–107.

Munroe, B., Smith, P. (1997) The value of a single structured bereavement visit. *British Journal of Community Health Nursing*. 2(5): 225–228.

National Institute for Clinical Excellence (2004) *Improving Supportive and Palliative Care for Adults with Cancer*. London: DoH.

Olieviere, D., Hargreaves, R., Monroe, B. (1998) *Good Practices in Palliative Care*. Aldergate: Ashgate.

Parkes, C.M. (1981) The evaluation of a bereavement service. *Journal of Preventative Psychiatry*. 1: 179–88.

Parkes, CM (2007) Dangerous words. *Bereavement Care* 26(2): 23–25.

Parkes, C.M. (2000) 'Bereavement as a psychological transition: processes of adaptation to change' in Dickenson, D., Johnson, M., Katz, J.S. (eds) *Death Dying & Bereavement*. London: Sage.

Parkes, C.M. (1998) Coping with loss: bereavement in adult life. *British Medical Journal*. 316: 856–859.

Stroebe, M. (1992) Coping with bereavement: a review of the grief work hypothesis. *Omega*. 40: 351–374.

Stroebe, M.S., Schut, M. (1999) 'The dual process model of coping with bereavement: rationale & description' *Death Studies*. 23: 197–224.

Thompson, N. (2012) *Grief and its challenges*. Basingstoke: Palgrave Macmillan.

Walsh, H.C. (2008a) Caring for bereaved people 1: models of bereavement. *Nursing Times*. 103 (51): 26–27.

Walsh, H.C. (2008b) Caring for bereaved people 2: nursing management. *Nursing Times,* 104 (1): 32–33.

Walter, T. (1997) Letting go and keeping hold: a reply to Stroebe. *Mortality*. 2(3): 263–66.

Walter, T. (1996) 'A new model of grief: bereavement biography' *Mortality*. 1 (1): 7–25.

Worden, W. (1982) *Grief Counselling and Grief Therapy: A Handbook for the Mental Health Practitioner*. New York: Springer.

Worden, J.W. (2010) *Greif Counselling and Grief Therapy: A Handbook for the Mental Health Practitioner*, 4th edn. Hove: Routledge.

III

Personal and professional development in palliative care

15

Looking after yourself

Introduction

Caring for and responding to the holistic needs of patients receiving palliative care and their families requires a whole person response. Giving of oneself in this way is demanding and requires the individual to take care of himself or herself. As long ago as the late 1990s, successive governments have recognised the need for staff working in the National Health Service (NHS) to look after themselves. Stotter (1992) suggests that the quality of care given to patients relies on the extent to which those caring for them feel cared for, if we feel well supported, then we are more able to support others. Whilst employing organisations do have a duty of care to ensure that their staff are supported, each individual also has a responsibility to care for himself or herself.

This chapter explores the reasons why self care is important. It explores the impact of stress along with its physical, psychological and behavioural manifestations and coping mechanisms before looking at formal and informal means of support.

Fundamentals of Palliative Care for Student Nurses, First Edition. Megan Rosser and Helen C. Walsh.

Companion website: www.wiley.com/go/rosser_walsh/fundamentals_of_palliative_care

Learning outcomes

By the end of this chapter you should be able to

- discuss the reasons why stress is prevalent in health care and palliative care in particular;
- define stress and recognise its manifestations;
- identify your own responses and coping mechanisms to stress;
- discuss formal and informal means of support.

Activity 15.1

Think about what stress means to you. You may find it helpful to consider developing a mind map.

What is stress and why do we need to know about it?

Palmer (1989) defines stress as the psychological, physiological and behavioural response by an individual when they perceive a lack of equilibrium between the demands placed upon them and their ability to meet those demands, which, over a period of time, leads to ill health. Put more simply, stress can be considered as an imbalance between the demands facing an individual and the resources available to meet them. This leaves the individual feeling unable to cope with all that they have to do. Prolonged stress causes physical, mental and psychological harm which is distressing for the individual and could also be detrimental to patient care (Murray, 2005). Fact Box 15.1 shows some of the consequences of stress for the NHS.

Fact Box 15.1

Consequences of stress for the NHS

- Stress costs the NHS up to £530 million per annum (HSE, 2007).
- Stress accounts for around 30% of all NHS sickness.
- Sixty percent of NHS organisations believed that up to fifty percent of their staff experienced stress (Bruce, 2006).
- In 2008 sick days due to stress and its associated psychiatric problems accounted for 4% of all sick days in non-NHS organisations (Clews, 2009).
- In 2008 sick days due to stress and its associated psychiatric problems accounted for 15% of all sick days in NHS organisations (Clews, 2009).

Fact Box 15.2

Physical symptoms of stress

Palpitations, sweating, increase in blood pressure, sweaty palms, tightness in chest/throat/shoulders, aching neck/jaw/ back muscles, muscle tenseness, repeated swallowing, dry mouth, heavy lethargic feelings, indigestion, tingling in the arms/back of neck, general aches/pains, sniffing, wobbly knees, blushing, squeaky voice, acne, shivering, cold hands/feet, changes in eating/sleeping patterns/bowel habits, headaches, migraines, chest pains, abdominal cramps, nausea, stomach aches, restlessness, flushing, shallow breathing, trembling, sleep disturbances, tiredness, itching, susceptibility to minor illness, easily startled, forgetfulness, menstrual problems, breathlessness, fast breathing, wanting to pass urine, visual disturbances, exhaustion, feeling cold/faint, frequent colds, loss of libido.

Fact Box 15.3

Behavioural responses to stress

Withdrawal, lack of socialising, under or over eating/alcohol/drugs/nicotine/gambling, poor timekeeping, less attention to diet, health, hygiene, becoming accident prone, careless, becoming impatient, aggressive or compulsive, pacing, fidgeting, swearing, blaming, throwing, hitting, working longer, foregoing breaks, taking work home, poor time management, 'headless chicken' syndrome, no time for leisure activities, outbursts, gripping something tightly, loss of interest, manic behaviour, unnecessary risks, illogical behaviour, increased sick time/working when sick, useless activity, nail biting, picking fights.

Fact Box 15.4

Cognitive and emotional responses to stress

Mind racing/going blank, not being able to switch off, lack of attention to detail, lowered self-esteem/confidence, disorganised thoughts, diminished sense of meaning to life, lack of control, need for too much control, negative self statements and evaluation, difficulty making decisions, loss of perspective 'making mountains out of molehills', driving yourself too hard, thought blocks, lack of concentration, suppression of feelings, 'What's the matter with me, everyone else copes?' self doubt, procrastination, hopelessness, shutting out thoughts, over-intellectualising, missing the point, not being able to see wood for the trees, fear of thinking for yourself, escapism, hypercritical, irrational, irritability, anger, depression, jealousy, restlessness, anxiety, unreal or hyper alert, unnecessary guilt, panic, mood swings, crying easily, hysteria, bewilderment, feeling sorry for oneself, emotionally cold, helplessness, feeling unworthy, despair, feeling stupid, vulnerability, feelings of inadequacy, euphoria, feeling lonely, sense of losing control, hurt, deflation, sadness, worry, moodiness.

Whilst it is important to understand the wider consequences of stress, the focus of this chapter is on looking after yourself and consequently the need to understand how stress affects you.

Activity 15.2

Think about a situation which you know you found stressful. How did you react physically and emotionally? What did you think and how did you behave?

Compare your responses to those identified in the following fact boxes (adapted from the work of Bond 1986; Murray, 2005; Lambert and Lambert, 2008).

Stress can manifest itself in an emotional, physical or psychological manner and all three may be present at the same time. All the symptoms listed above however, can also be the result of other psychological or physical conditions and Lambert and Lambert (2008) recommend that someone experiencing stress should visit their GP to rule out any underlying medical or psychological condition.

Whilst stress can be detrimental to our health, some stress is necessary to help us perform.

Consider the diagrams in Figures 15.1 and 15.2.

These diagrams illustrate that too little pressure and stress can be as bad for us as too much. Whilst you might be happy and content for the first few days of a holiday to just lie by the pool soaking up the sun, at some point you will become bored. Similarly, a really busy shift presenting loads of challenges maybe exciting and stimulating at first, but if the pace continues day after day at some point you will become over stimulated, leading to fatigue and exhaustion. The tipping point is different for everybody and often it rests on our perception of the stressors.

Stressors are outside pressures which contribute to the body experiencing a physiological stress reaction, involving complex metabolic, endocrine, cardiovascular and neurological responses. If this response continues over a long period of time ill health and burnout will result. A definition of burnout can be found in Fact Box 15.5.

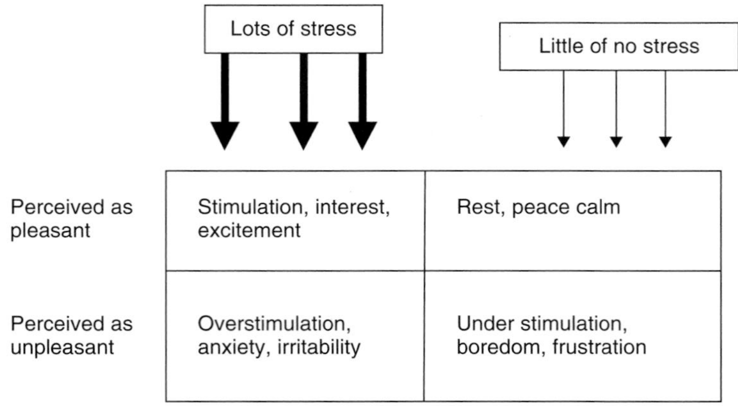

Figure 15.1 Perceptions of stress.

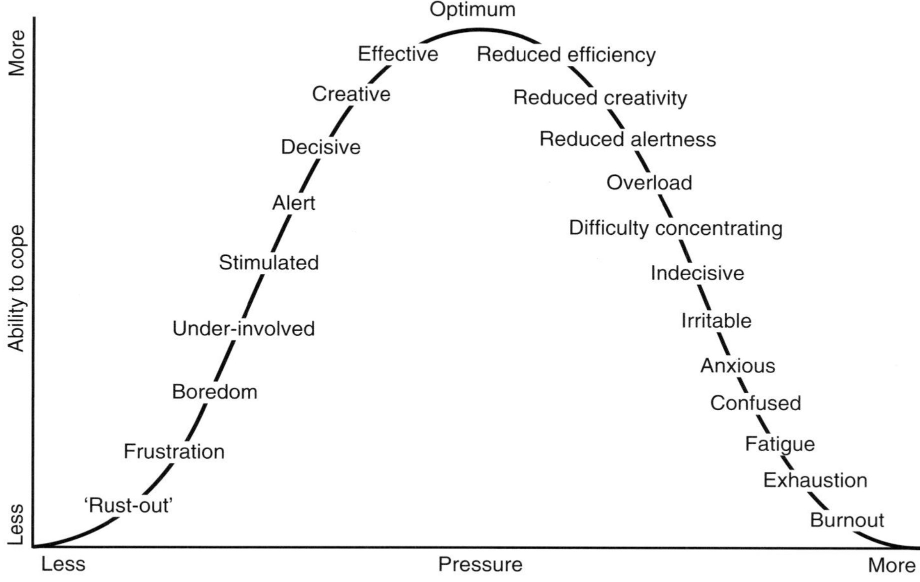

Figure 15.2 The effects of different levels of stress.

Fact Box 15.5

Burnout defined

Maslech and Jackson (1981) define burnout as a physical, emotional and intellectual exhaustion syndrome manifested by an adverse attitude to professional life and other people with the development of a negative self-esteem in the individual experiencing chronic fatigue and feelings of helplessness and hopelessness.

Evidence of burnout may be manifested in maladaptive nursing behaviours such as disengagement, avoidance of meaningful contact with patients/families, blocking communication techniques and sarcasm/negative appraisal/defeatism.

Activity 15.3

Think about your life working as a student nurse. What makes it stressful for you? You might like to use a mind map to record your thoughts. Now think about working with patients receiving palliative care. What makes this stressful for you? Add your answers to your mind map. You may have identified some of the issues discussed below.

Some of the reasons nursing is stressful

Nursing is often stressful, as is caring for patients with palliative care needs, often for similar reasons. Lambert and Lambert (2008), Setch (2001) and Suresh *et al.* (2012) identify that these stressors come from many sources including:

- our feelings
  - that we lack the necessary confidence and competency;
  - fear of making a mistake;
  - being isolated from other students and experiencing loneliness;
  - discomfort with the intimacy and close physical contact involved in nursing;
  - lack of support from colleagues;
  - frustration of expectations, not living up to reality.
- inadequate skills – be they technical or effective interpersonal skills, necessary when dealing with patients from diverse backgrounds, often with complex needs;
- caring for patients who have been exposed to gross trauma, injury, have undergone mutilating surgery or experiencing severe and intense pain; within palliative care, patients may also experience other intractable and distressing symptoms such as breathlessness, nausea and vomiting;

- dealing with
  - sensitive issues such as body image, sexuality;
  - role conflict;
  - student status;
  - chaotic environments;
  - hierarchical structures.
- having to be flexible and versatile to deal with the challenges of practice, for example, the unexpected, the inappropriate, shift changes;
- balancing academic, practice and family demands;
- frequently joining and leaving established nursing teams to gain different clinical experiences;
- too much responsibility;
- excessive workload;
- challenging working relationships;
- lack of resources and/or people.

In addition to these stressors above, working in palliative care has additional challenges. For example, whilst dying and death are not exclusive to palliative care, they are part of everyday practice and generally spoken of more openly. This can often raise ethical dilemmas when considering what information to give to patients and their families, do you tell them the whole truth, some of the truth or withhold information? Patients receiving palliative care may have experienced significant changes to their self image as a result of the disease itself, such as a fungating wound, or the consequence of treatment which can cause challenges in building therapeutic relationships.

Effects of stress

Activity 15.4

What do you think are the consequences of long-term stress on both the individual and the nursing team? Compare your answers with those in Table 15.1.

Table 15.1 The effects of stress on the individual and the health care team.

Individual	Team
Poor relationships with patients	Poor team-working
Poor relationships with peers/colleagues	Poor communication
Errors of judgement	Increased staff turnover
Poor practice/communication	Increased sickness/absence
Increased risk taking	Impaired continuity of care
Demotivation	Poor quality of care
Lack of job satisfaction	Decision making in isolation
Lack of commitment	Low morale

Coping strategies

If we are facing stress, then we have to develop ways of coping with it. Coping reflects the changes we make to our thoughts and behaviours in an effort to manage the internal or external demands that we consider to be taxing or exceeding our resources. Coping strategies, as the name suggests, are the strategies or approaches we use to help change our thoughts and behaviours, so that we can use our resources more effectively to cope with the stress.

Activity 15.5

Spend some time thinking about your own coping strategies. What helps you manage the stress you experience in work and also the stresses you have outside work? How effective are they? Is there anything else you could consider using?

Basically a strategy can be anything that works for you. Whilst something might be effective it does not necessarily mean that it is good for us. It might be very effective in the short term, but detrimental over long periods of time. How easy might it be for that glass of wine, after a particularly hard shift, to become a glass every evening? And then, for that glass to get bigger, as we need more to have the same effect?

Coping strategies are usually something we use consistently because they have helped us in the past. Coping strategies can be considered under three headings: defence mechanisms, emotion focused and problem focussed (Lambert and Lambert, 2008).

Defence mechanisms are psychological strategies brought into play by the unconscious mind in order to manipulate, deny, or distort reality enabling the individual to see the situation differently (Barker, 2007). They protect the individual from anxiety, social sanctions and provide a refuge from a situation which the individual finds difficulty coping with. By changing unacceptable stimuli or impulses into something which is acceptable, the unconscious blocks them out, thus reducing anxiety. Whilst there is no agreement on exactly how many defence mechanisms there are (Barker, 2007), the main ones are briefly described in Table 15.2.

Table 15.2 Defence mechanisms.

Mechanism	Description
Denial	Used unconsciously to resolve emotional conflict and anxiety, the unpleasant aspects of a situation which are uncomfortable or painful are denied. The reality maybe denied altogether (simple denial), its seriousness minimised (its not that bad) or when both the fact and seriousness are acknowledged, responsibility is denied (it was not my fault).
Displacement	The mind redirects emotion from a 'dangerous' to a 'safe' object. For example, you may have looked after a patient who was very rude to you; obviously it would be unprofessional to be rude back, so when you finish your shift you may shout at your partner. Most often, we take out our frustrations on the people we love.
Intellectualisation	Involves removing oneself from the situation by concentrating on the intellectual aspects, hiding emotions and feelings behind facts and big words. For example, a wife whose husband is dying may try to learn everything about his disease and talk about it in scientific terms, describing the medical facts about his condition. In doing so she protects herself from the distress of acknowledging that her husband is dying.
Projection	This involves attributing to others one's own undesirable thoughts and/or emotions. For example, you may not like your friend's new partner, Alex, but your unconscious mind won't allow you acknowledge this. Instead of admitting your dislike, you 'project' it onto Alex and your conscious thought is not 'I don't like Alex' but rather 'Alex doesn't like me'.
Rationalisation	A process of constructing a logical justification for a decision that was originally arrived at through a different mental process, that is, making excuses for own mistakes or disappointments, avoiding self-condemnation

	or condemnation by others. 'Sour grapes' rationalisation explains away the disappointment of not getting the hoped for practice placement by saying 'I wouldn't have liked it anyway' whilst 'silver lining' rationalisation recognises that 'I now have the opportunity to work elsewhere'.
Reaction formation	Involves anxiety-producing or unacceptable emotions being replaced by their direct opposites. For example, one who is strongly in favour of euthanasia, but has moral, religious or professional obligations to avoid it, might become a staunch critic. In this way there is no threat from or even an awareness of, the emotion.
Regression	Involves returning to a point in time when we felt safe and secure. Our behaviour may become more childish and primitive as we try to relate to the world in a way that was formerly effective, giving up mature problem solving methods of dealing with challenges.
Repression/ Suppression	Both mechanisms involving pulling painful or dangerous thoughts into the unconscious, preventing them entering consciousness. Whilst repression is an unconscious force, suppression is a conscious process, that is, a conscious choice not to think about something
Sublimation	Refocusing energy away from negative to more positive outlets. For example, many great charities were started by people whose loved ones either died or suffered from a disease or disability.
Compensation	Recognising a weakness in one area and trying to excel in another is a healthy way to handle the anxiety of feeling inferior or inadequate. There are unhealthy ways to compensate, such as a person feeling unloved becoming promiscuous, substituting quantity for quality.
Dissociation	Usually originates after a trauma, intense pain or a period of prolonged intense stress and may manifest itself as flashbacks or forgetting something embarrassing or in more serious disorders such as Post-Traumatic Stress Disorder. Memories are lost in the subconscious becoming splintered and distorted. A person may remember what happened, but forget how it felt.
Fantasy	A way to escape real problems. Imagining that one is successful may lead to feelings of success. However, imagining the worst consequences may lead to fear, and reliving a bad situation may lead to anger and depression.
Identification	Involves taking on someone else's personal characteristics, in order to solve some emotional difficulty and avoid anxiety.
Undoing	Based on the notion that it is possible to make amends, it involves feeling guilty and trying to do something to undo the harm that may have been inflicted.
Withdrawal	Involves the removal of oneself from anything and everything that carries reminders of painful or stressful thoughts and emotions.

There are two main ways a person uses defence mechanisms to cope with threats:

- avoiding stress using defence mechanisms such as repression, denial, withdrawal and projection. This approach reduces stress by avoiding the situation and can be very effective when the situation is outside our control.
- approaching the situation using defence mechanisms such as rationalisation, identification and compensation. The individual seeks to learn more about the situation and tries to take charge which works well when there is something that can be done.

Depending on the situation, most people use both approaches, although they tend to have a preferred way of dealing with the stress. Each has its own disadvantages, the 'approachers' tend to experience more stress and worry and the 'avoiders' continue to lack awareness.

Activity 15.6

Consider the coping mechanisms listed in Table 15.2 and see if any of them are similar to your own ways of coping. How effective do you find them?

Whilst useful in the short term, prolonged use of defence mechanisms can separate the individual from reality and their true feelings. This may explain why nurses sometimes experience 'burnout' or appear unmoved when faced with distressing situations.

In addition to using defence mechanisms to help us cope, we also use emotion focussed or problem focussed strategies. Emotion focussed coping strategies (Box 15.1) involve the individual trying to directly moderate or eliminate unpleasant emotions. They do this through activities such as using humour, attempting to keeping things normal, maintaining routine or talking. Aiming to short circuit negative emotions, problem focussed coping strategies (Box 15.1) attempt to modify, avoid or minimise the threat. With both approaches, behaviour is changed

Box 15.1 Stress relieving strategies

Emotion focussed strategies	**Problem focussed strategies**
Seeking social and emotional support	Seeking information about what to do
Distancing – making cognitive efforts to detach from situation	Holding back from impulsive and premature actions
Escape – wishful thinking or escaping/avoiding situation through sleeping or drugs	Confronting the person or persons responsible for one's difficulty
Self-control – attempts to modulate feelings or actions regarding the problem	
Accepting responsibility – acknowledging own role in the problem	
Positive reappraisal – creating a positive meaning in terms of personal growth	

to deal with the stress. It is possible to use these strategies independently or together depending on the situation.

Consider Lucy, a third year nursing student and how she copes with her workload. Lucy is nearing the end of her degree studies. She is currently on her management placement in an inpatient hospice unit. The unit has been particularly busy lately as a number of younger people have been admitted with advanced disease. Alongside the stress of the work place, Lucy is also preparing for important examinations. Lucy employs the following mechanisms to help her cope.

Lucy organises a study group with her friends from college so that together they can go over the course material in a systematic way, learning from and helping each other **(problem-focused coping)**. Before going for this meeting Lucy recognises that she has to relax and collect her thoughts together, so takes a long hot bath **(emotion-focused coping)**. Following the meeting Lucy decides that she needs to develop an action plan **(problem-focused coping)**, but before she settles down to any work she spends an hour or so watching her favourite 'soaps' on television **(emotion-focused coping)**.

Managing your stress

When it comes to managing your stress there are basically two approaches to reduce the amount of stress or to increase our ability to deal with it as highlighted in Box 15.1. There are three levels of managing stress. Level 1 involves you becoming aware of what stresses you. Because the experience of stress depends to a large extent on your perception of it, you need to be an expert in managing your own stress. You need to know what stresses you, the effect it has on you, what coping mechanisms you currently use and how effective they are. Where necessary you might need to review your lifestyle, adopting much more effective coping mechanisms if necessary. It is easy to talk about managing your personal and work environments, but many aspects of these areas are beyond your control. If you can alter aspects of the situation then you should seek to do so, but you also need to develop the ability to accept the things you cannot change. You do need to reprogramme your thinking to try and ignore the negative and focus on the positive.

Level 2 requires you to identify personal solutions for managing stress and putting them into practice. This could involve seeking structured channels for relaxation, for example, aromatherapy and appropriate physical and emotional outlets. More information is shown Box 15.2. Level 3 is reserved for formal activities such as clinical supervision, counselling and when the stress is severe, medical interventions.

Another approach to managing stress is prioritisation. This involves you identifying:

- **What you MUST do?**
- **What you SHOULD do?**
- **What you COULD do?**

You need to review this list regularly because what might be a 'could' today might become a 'should' or even a 'must' by next week. So for example, consider two activities: meeting up with a friend and preparing an assignment. With the submission date a month away, working on the assignment is something that you could do whereas meeting the friend is something you feel that you must do. With two weeks to go before submission, you should do both, whilst the night before submission, you must work on the assignment, although you could meet the friend.

Box 15.2 Actions and solutions for managing stress

Action	Solutions
Avoid unnecessary stress	Learn to say 'no' Avoid people who do not make you feel good Avoid controversial topics Keep a reasonable 'to-do list'
Alter the situation	Express your feelings Be willing to compromise Be more assertive Develop time management skills
Accept the things that you cannot change	Do not try to control the uncontrollable See the positive Forgive
Adapt to the stressor	Try and look at problems differently Try and see the big picture Re-evaluate your standards Focus on the positive
Address your personal needs	Have 'me' time Spend time with friends who make you feel good Do something every day that is enjoyable Exercise regularly Laugh often Eat healthily Avoid alcohol, smoking and drugs

Setch (2001) advises us firstly to identify where we get our support and specifically the people who make us feel supported. She advises us to think about the different situations in which we might need support and then identify the people who provide the appropriate support.

Activity 15.7

Read the types of support identified below and try and identify a person (or persons) who is there for you at those times identified.

1. **When you need to be accepted** – you need someone who listens in a non-judgmental way and resists from giving you advice.
   The person I turn to is
2. **When you need personal support –** unconditional support even though they may not agree with what you say or what you want to do.
   The person I turn to is

3. **When you need to be challenged on a personal level** – you need someone who can ask you incisive questions whilst checking out your thoughts, feelings and behaviour.
   The person I turn to is
4. **When you need support and challenge related to work** – you need someone who knows your job and can help you identify your strengths and cope the difficulties.
   The person I turn to is
5. **When you need support during times of crisis** – you need a professional who can listen to you, for example, counsellor, occupational health nurse.
   The person I turn to is

(Adapted from Setch, 2001.)

Whilst some people may be able to help you in more than one area, it is not good to rely too much on them. If you have found that one or two names have cropped up in more than one category, you may need to think about identifying someone else to help in one of the areas. It is often better and more effective to have personal and work support from different people as they offer different perspectives.

The above activity has focussed on identifying the people who you find supportive. Whilst it is worthwhile having people to help you, we each have our own support strategies which we use frequently to help us cope with the stresses of life. These can range from walking the dog, going to the gym, shopping or socialising.

Activity 15.8

Spend some time thing about the support strategies you use. You might not have consciously thought about the things you do as being 'supportive' before, so you may come back to this list as you realise that something you do actually helps you cope better. Consider the activities under the following headings:

Activity;
Frequency;
How pleasurable is it?
How effective do you find it?

Activity 15.9

When you have completed Activities 15.7 and 15.8, what do you make of your support mechanisms? Do they work for you? Do you need to make some adjustments, add more people, plug some gaps, make adjustments? How will you do this?

Setch (2001) goes on to talk about 'The Support Menu' which she describes as consisting of a starter, main course and dessert. Starters consists of those activities you do by yourself, the main courses are those activities you do with colleagues such as reflective practice, education and training, and desserts are activities you do with others but away from work environment such as a social event or aromatherapy. As with a restaurant menu, sometimes we only need one course, sometimes two and at other times we go the whole hog and have the lot. It is up to us to choose depending on our circumstances at that time. The same principles apply with the support menu. The options we have, the greater our choice to 'mix and match,' so the support we access matches our needs.

Conclusion

It is important that we remember to look after ourselves. Nursing and working with patients and families receiving palliative care involves us taking on others pain, emotions, anxieties and fears. Nurses see and experience events and situations which are often very difficult and challenging physically and emotionally. Supporting others is costly for ourselves and we in turn require and deserve support. Long-term unmanaged stress is harmful, both for the individual and also potentially for the patient. Each of us has coping strategies. Good adaptive coping strategies are helpful and have no long-term side effects and whilst others are immediately effective, they may be associated with long-term risks. We need to identify what stresses us and how we cope with it, making appropriate changes to ensure we receive safe, effective support. Mark Twain said 'If you always do what you always did, you'll always get what you've always got' and Einstein said 'Only the insane carry on doing the same thing and expect different results'. If our coping mechanisms and means of support are ineffective, carrying on will mean we do not manage stress effectively.

Glossary

Aromatherapy	A form of complimentary therapy-uses plant essential oils for the purpose of altering a person's mood, cognitive function or health.
Burnout	A psychological term for a syndrome characterised by long-term exhaustion and diminished interest, particularly in one's work and career.
Chemotherapy	The treatment of cancer with one or more cytotoxic antineoplastic drugs as part of a standardised regime.
Continuity of care	The degree to which care is coherent and linked.
Coping	The process of managing stressful circumstances.
Coping strategies	Activities, behaviours or rituals which help the process of managing stressful circumstances.
Defence mechanisms	Psychological strategies brought into play by the unconscious mind to manipulate, distort or deny reality in order to protect the individual from feelings of anxiety.

Demotivation	A feeling of disillusionment, disinclination to be involved or productive in the work setting.
Equilibrium	The condition within a person or a situation where all competing influences are balanced.
Escapism	Mental diversion by means of entertainment or recreation used as an 'escape' from perceived unpleasant stimuli of life.
Ethical dilemma	A complex situation that often involves mental conflict between moral imperatives where to obey one, transgresses another.
Hypercritical	Making harsh judgements of one's actions, behaviour or thoughts.
Job satisfaction	The level to which an individual is satisfied with his or her job.
Lethargy	A subjective feeling of tiredness.
Migraine	A chronic neurological disorder characterised by recurrent moderate to severe headaches often accompanied by a range of autonomic nervous system symptoms.
Over-intellectualising	The process of 'over thinking' a situation in order to avoid painful or distressing emotions.
Palpitations	An abnormality of the heart beat ranging from unnoticed skipped beats or accelerated heart rate to very noticeable changes accompanied by dizziness and breathlessness.
Perception	The organisation, identification and interpretation of sensory information in order for the individual to understand the environment.
Procrastination	Deliberately putting off impending tasks and doing other less important or more enjoyable ones.
Prolonged stress	The response to emotional pressure suffered for a long period of time over which the individual perceives they have no control.
Psychiatric problems	A range of psychological patterns of behaviours, feelings, thoughts generally associated with distress or disability which are not considered part of the normal development in a individual's culture.
Radiotherapy	The medical use of ionising radiation as part of cancer treatment to control or kill malignant cells.

Reflective practice The process of thinking about practice in order to learn and develop as a professional.

Self image The mental picture a person holds about themselves based on factual information such has height, hair colour and from personal experience and internalising the judgments of others.

Staff turnover The rate at which staff join and leave a place of work.

Stress A feeling of strain and pressure which is often accompanied by a range of emotional and physical manifestations.

Stressor A chemical or biological agent, environmental condition, external stimulus or event that causes stress to an individual.

Therapeutic relationship The relationship between a nurse and patient where both engage with each other in the hope of bringing about a positive change for the patient.

References

Barker, S. (2007). *Psychology.* Oxford: Blackwell Publishing.

Bond, M. (1986). *Stress & Self-Awareness: A Guide for Nurses*. Oxford: Heinemann Nursing.

Bruce, M. (2006). Say goodbye to stress. *Nursing Standard*. 20(22): P72.

Clew G (2009). NHS stress driving up nurse sick leave levels. Nursing Times.net available at http://www.nursingtimes.net/nursing-practice/clinical-zones/occupational-health/nhs-stress-driving-up-nurse-sick-leave-levels/5000401.article

HSE 2007 workplace stress costs Great Britain in excess of £530 million available at: http://www.hse.gov.uk/press/2007/c07021.htm.

Lambert, V.A. and Lambert, C.E. (2008). Nurses' workplace stressors and coping strategies. *Indian Journal of Palliative Care*. 14(1): 38–44.

Maslech, C. and Jackson, S.E. (1981). The measurement of experienced burnout. *Journal of Occupational Behaviour*. 2: 99–113.

Palmer, S. (1989). Occupational stress. *The Health & Safety Practitioner*. 7(8): 16–18.

Murray, R. (2005). *Managing Your Stress A Guide for Nurses.* London: RCN.

Setch, F. (2001). Looking after yourself. In: Kinghorn, S. and Gamlin, R. (eds). *Palliative Nursing Bringing Comfort and Hope*. London: Balliere Tindall, Chapter 17.

Stotter, D. (1992). The culture of care. *Nursing Times.* 88(12): 30–31.

Suresh, P., Matthews, A. and Coyne, I. (2012). Stress and stressors in the clinical environment: a comparative study of fourth year student nurses and newly qualified general nurses in Ireland. *Journal of Clinical Nursing*. 22: 770–779.

16

Professional support

Introduction

Working in health care is extremely rewarding, but can be very stressful, often because it takes place within the context of significant human suffering (Aranda, 2008). Caring for patients and families receiving palliative care brings its own unique rewards and stresses. Both patient and family are often distressed, experiencing pain, either emotional or psychological, and struggling to come to terms with existential questions of meaning (Aranda, 2008). Palliative care can be emotionally demanding and without adequate support or training can exact a considerable cost (McVey and Jones, 2012). We all get out of our depth at times, feeling overwhelmed by the things we see, the patients and families we nurse and the situations we face. We need to become self-aware, recognising our strengths, resources and limitations. Part of this process involves us knowing when and where to get additional help and support.

The Royal College of Nursing (RCN) (2011) suggests considering accessing support from colleagues, the chaplaincy or psychological team, local contacts specific for the workplace and appropriate faith groups or support networks. This chapter explores the benefits of support from some of these sources.

Fundamentals of Palliative Care for Student Nurses, First Edition. Megan Rosser and Helen C. Walsh.

Companion website: www.wiley.com/go/rosser_walsh/fundamentals_of_palliative_care

Learning outcomes

By the end of this chapter you should be able to

- recognise the role of professional support;
- discuss the importance of key people in providing support;
- identify key components of clinical supervision.

Key people

There are a number of key people who can offer you support and in this section we will briefly discuss the roles of four of them. They are the personal tutor, clinical mentor, occupational health department and student services.

Personal tutor

Your personal tutor is likely to be a constant throughout your time in the University. The specific role of the personal tutor varies between different universities and among other things they may offer academic and pastoral support. Sometimes, as students, issues or problems may develop in your personal lives or within clinical practice, which may then impact on each other and on academic studies. The personal tutor is in a position to help support you through these difficulties, often by helping you understand and attend to their impact on clinical practice and your academic studies. For example, extensions for assignment submission dates and changes in placements. Always remember that your personal tutor cannot help if they are unaware of what is happening to you.

Your relationship with your personal tutor is an important and professional relationship. As such, personal preferences should not be an issue. Sometimes, however, personality clashes occur. If you feel you are unable to relate to the personal tutor you have been allocated, seek to change this. Your University should have a policy to help you do this.

Mentor

While in clinical practice, you will be allocated a mentor and the RCN (2011) acknowledges that the mentor should serve as a source of trustworthy support. Over time the word 'mentor' has come to mean a designated person who gives time to help individuals learn during their developmental years. The concept and practice of mentorship to facilitate professional development in health care has evolved consistently since the 1970s (Gopee, 2011) and was formally implemented into pre-registration nurse education in the 1980s (United Kingdom Central Council for Nursing Midwifery and Health Visiting, 1986). Within nurse education, the mentor fulfils a formal role providing support and assessment of competence in order to enable nursing students to gain safe and effective clinical skills during placements.

The role of mentor lacks a clear and universally accepted definition. There are, however, numerous agreed 'helper' functions involved in the role including advisor, teacher, role model and assessor (Morton-Cooper and Palmer, 2000; Nursing and Midwifery Council (NMC) 2008).

Box 16.1 NMC expectations of a mentor

Supporting students in identifying their learning needs and helping them gain experience appropriate to their level of learning.

Using a range of learning experiences, including patients and the Multi-disciplinary team (MDT) to meet define needs.

Acting as a resource to facilitate personal and professional development of others, including nursing students.

The NMC (2008) suggests that mentoring is the giving of support, assistance and guidance to learning new skills, adopting new behaviours and acquiring new attitudes. Within nursing, it is now a mandatory requirement that pre-registration nursing students are supported and assessed by mentors who fulfil specific criteria relating to experience, training and qualifications (NMC, 2008). The mentor is responsible for organising and coordinating learning activities in practice, which involve supervising students, providing constructive feedback, assessing total performance and providing evidence for achievement of competence (NMC, 2008). A nurse mentor is, therefore, an experienced registered nurse who helps learners apply the theoretical knowledge they have to real-life situations and who is also responsible for assessing clinical competence and professional behaviour (Bennett, 2002). The NMC (2008) expectations of a mentor are shown in Box 16.1.

As a nursing student you are an adult learner and to some extent must be prepared to take responsibility for your own learning about palliative care. You need to know in advance where your placement is in order to give you time to prepare and to identify possible learning goals, particularly in relation to palliative care that you wish to discuss with your mentor. Your mentor can help you develop an action plan which should detail specific learning objectives with some idea of how they are to be achieved. The more specific these are, the more easily you will identify what you have learnt and be able to recognise your own development in palliative care.

The mentor has a crucial role in supporting students to learn about palliative care. It is their responsibility to see that the student is able to undertake supervised and appropriately guided experience to develop and practice palliative nursing skills. Palliative care is often a dynamic and rapidly changing environment and any situation may present a learning opportunity. Cross (2009) recognises that the presence of a prepared and competent mentor will facilitate and maximise opportunistic learning. With continuous support and frequent meetings, the mentor can enable the student to explore their own personal feelings and emotions by structuring discussions around areas of palliative care that the student may encounter. It is also an opportunity to review clinical skills such as communication and symptom control.

Activity 16.1

Consider your clinical placements to date and the various mentors you have worked with. What clinical skills have they helped you develop? How have they helped you develop professionally? What about personally?

Activity 16.2

Either:

Think about times when you have nursed patients receiving palliative care. With hindsight, what do you think were your learning needs and your support needs? How did your mentor help to facilitate your learning and provide you with support?

Or:

Imagine you are going to be caring for patients receiving palliative care. What do you think your learning needs are and what support do you think you might need? How do you think your mentor can help to facilitate your learning and support you?

Mentors can provide support through facilitating learning using either formal or informal activities (Gopee, 2011). Formal activities include direct teaching, setting learning tasks and enabling students to spend time with doctors, other members of the multi-disciplinary team and attending relevant meetings and case conferences. Informal activities include allowing students to talk to patients and their families, making time for informal chats and 'debriefing' as well as facilitating individual reflection.

University Services

Student services

The University will have a department dedicated to supporting students, providing advice on a range of issues, counselling, help with academic skills and, in some cases, financial advice and support. It is worth finding out what your particular student services offer so that you know where to go if you need to.

The occupational health department

The University has an occupational health department staffed by specially trained health care staff. These can offer help with health issues, including stress, and provide a confidential service.

Clinical supervision

Clinical supervision has been suggested as the answer to many of the challenges facing nursing today (Bishop, 2008a, 2008b). This is a very bold claim about a concept which is often misunderstood and sometimes misused.

What is clinical supervision?

The term supervision conjures up various thoughts and feelings, depending on the individual's experiences and opinions (Cassedy, 2010). These can often result in a feeling of hostility towards supervision and a fear of one's practice coming under close scrutiny. These fears are unjustified if clinical supervision is organised and undertaken appropriately.

The origins of clinical supervision lie within the field of mental health nursing and until the 1990s was an activity undertaken by the elite few (Bishop, 2006). In 1994, the Department of Health commissioned a review of clinical supervision, resulting in the publication of a position paper (Faugier and Butterworth, 1994). This was widely circulated throughout the National Health Service (NHS) and the independent sector accompanied by a letter from the Chief Nursing Officer. The letter declared that clinical supervision was fundamental to safeguarding standards and developing professional expertise in order to deliver quality care (DoH, 1994).

The reasons why clinical supervision moved into mainstream nursing include organisational instability, fast turn over, ever increasing workloads and advancing technology; these are still prevalent in the NHS and health care. Consequently, clinical supervision is still important today. Bishop (2008a) considers clinical supervision to be so important that nurses should be crying out for it and indeed refusing to work without it. Clinical supervision requires time and ideally should be part and parcel of the employment contract and if it is not, Fowler (2013) argues that it is so important that we should be prepared to engage in it in our own time. McVey and Jones (2012) maintain that providing clinical supervision should be seen as a measure of good practice within health care organisations.

In many ways clinical supervision is difficult to define as there is no one universally agreed definition or purpose. Table 16.1 shows some of the definitions which are contained in the literature.

Activity 16.3

Read the definitions listed in Table 16.1 and try and identify the common factors between them.

Your list of similarities between these very definitions should include the following:

- professional relationship;
- focus on professional issues;
- aimed to develop and review practice;
- regular meetings.

Why do we need clinical supervision?

Clinical supervision is not something that 'gets done' to us but is something that all practitioners can give and receive provided they share a common understanding of its purpose (Bishop, 2008b). Indeed, many professional organisations such as the NMC and the RCN view clinical supervision as essential (McVey and Jones, 2012). By its very nature, working in health care can often be stressful as it involves dealing with people who find themselves in many challenging and emotional situations. We are required to deliver high standards of care, continually improve our practice in order to ensure evidence-based care. We may often need support, help and guidance to achieve these goals, and clinical supervision is one mechanism which may help. McVey and Jones (2012) suggest that clinical supervision has a significant role to play in helping nurses develop and maintain the skills they need to continue to care for patients.

The opportunities offered by clinical supervision are shown in Box 16.2.

Table 16.1 Definitions of clinical supervision.

'An exchange between practising professionals to enable the development of professional skills, an opportunity to sustain and develop professional practice' (Butterworth and Faugier 1993).
A mechanism for improving the quality of patient care, maintaining and safeguarding standards of care, valuing the development of professional practice and knowledge (Bishop, 1994).
'A formal process of professional support and learning, which enables individual practitioners to develop knowledge and competence, assume responsibility for their own practice and enhance consumer protection and safety of care in complex clinical situations. It is central to the process of learning and to the expansion of the scope of practice and should be seen as the means for encouraging self-assessment and analytic and reflective skills' (DoH, 1993).
A practice-focussed, professional relationship to ensure high quality nursing practice and care to patients, and to provide support to staff in their professional role (Northern Health and Social Services Board, 1998 cited by Bishop, 2008a, 2008b).
A practice-focused professional relationship that enables you to reflect on your practice with the support of a skilled supervisor. Through reflection you can further develop your skills, knowledge and enhance your understanding of your own practice (NMC, 2005).
Clinical supervision is an effective way of providing staff with support, while developing and maintaining their communication and psychological skills (Mannix *et al.*, 2006).
Clinical supervision is a designated interaction between two or more practitioners within a safe and supportive environment that enables a continuum of reflective critical analysis of care to ensure quality patients services and the well-being of the practitioner (Bishop and Sweeney, 2006 cited by Bishop, 2008).
Clinical supervision can be defined as a regular and formal agreement to engage in a professional working relationship, facilitated by the supervisor to support the supervisee to reflect on practice, with the aim of developing quality care, accountability, personal competence and learning (Cassedy, 2010).
Clinical supervision involves spending time with a more experienced clinician, exploring what you do, how you do it and how you could do it better (Fowler, 2013).

Box 16.2 Opportunities of clinical supervision (Bishop, 2008b)

Clinical supervision offers:

emotional support, debriefing and nurturing through providing 'pit-head' time for us to wash off the dirt of practice (Hawkins and Shohet, 1989);

a buffer mechanism between harsh realities of practice and emotional/problem focused coping;
opportunity of critique from a peer or expert leading to professional growth and development;
space and time to reflect on one's work within a safe and trusting relationship.

Principles of clinical supervision

Whilst there are many definitions and models of clinical supervision, there are certain common principles. First, it is a formal system allowing practitioners to review clinical practice based on a mutually agreed contract between the supervisor and supervisee. The focus of the discussion is led by the supervisee, but both supervisor and supervisees have recognised rights and responsibilities (see Table 16.1). Supervision is aimed at improving and supporting practice so the focus should be on finding solutions to challenges and problems, and as a consequence, those involved should increase their understanding of professional issues. Whilst standards of care should be improved, clinical supervision also has the potential to increase practitioners' knowledge and skills and individuals should gain deeper and more insightful understanding of their own practice (NMC, 2006). Clinical supervision can occur as a group activity or as a one to one relationship. As long as those involved are committed to making it work, whichever format clinical supervision takes will meet the required needs.

Groups for clinical supervision can be closed, that is, once established no new members can join or open where attendance is on a drop in basis as and when required by the individual. Within group supervision, the supervisor can be one named individual or it can rotate around the members with a frequency that suits that group. There are no hard and fast rules and one approach is no more effective or beneficial than another. The important thing is that whatever structure is chosen, it suits the required purpose and meets the needs of the individuals concerned. The basis of clinical supervision is a relationship between supervisor and one or more people, the purpose of which is to focus on professional issues in order to support the individual and to develop practice. If it is done well, clinical supervision has the potential to transform nursing practice (Fowler, 2013).

A model for clinical supervision

Although there are numerous models for clinical supervision (Campbell, 2006), these are often developed as a response to specific needs. The RCN (2002) suggests a three pronged approach that is

- formative (educative) – looking at the 'how to' of practice. This can often be useful for people who are new in post;
- restorative (supportive) – helping to deal with the emotional reactions to practice;
- normative (managerial) –looking at quality and standards.

Originally described by Proctor (1986), the model is illustrated in Figure 16.1. Clinical supervision occurs where the three circles overlap. It is probable that during a supervisory

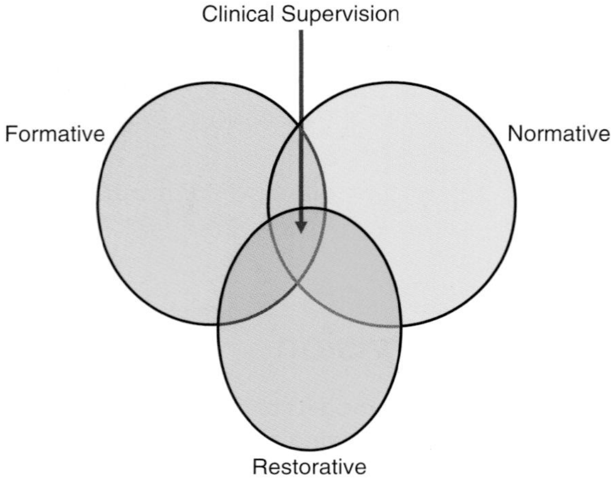

Clinical Supervision
Formative
Normative
Restorative

Figure 16.1 Proctor's model (1986).

relationship the focus will shift between the three areas, overall the balance should be equal to ensure that true clinical supervision is being provided. The crucial factor within clinical supervision is the relationship between the supervisor and the supervisee. It is essential that trust and respect exists between them for enabling the process of clinical supervision to be effective.

Benefits of clinical supervision

Unfortunately there are no clear and proven benefits of clinical supervision, although Cassedy (2010) identifies three potential beneficiaries which are listed in Box 16.3.

Box 16.3 Beneficiaries of clinical supervision (Cassedy, 2010)

The individual potentially benefits through

gaining learning opportunities and recognising the importance of lifelong learning;
identifying ways of integrating theory into practice;
reflecting on practice leading to improvements, increased confidence and competence;
increased self-awareness on personal and professional responsibilities and abilities;
increased support, motivation, creativity and staff support and morale;
validation and affirmation of ideas, views and feelings;
challenge and feedback, which in turns leads to new understanding and development.

The organisation potentially benefits through

safeguarding standards of care by promoting best practice through patient-focussed care planning;

promoting self-awareness and of professional accountability;

committed and motivated staff who are proactive within the organisation;

retention and recruitment of staff;

reduction in sickness rates.

Patients are likely to benefit through

all of the above leading to nursing care that is empathetic and ethically based provided by motivated nurses.

Butterworth *et al.* (2008) reviewed the literature published on clinical supervision in the United Kingdom between the years 2001–2007. Engagement in clinical supervision varied considerably, ranging from 18% of practice nurses in Leicestershire to almost 86% of mental health nurses in Northern Ireland. They found that the benefits of clinical supervision could be grouped together under three heading which were as follows.

Education and support

Used effectively, clinical supervision could be a device which resulted in growth and development of personality, increased confidence and self awareness, improved self care and work/life balance, improved relationships and a decrease in professional isolation. Clinical supervision also supports lifelong learning, leading to increased personal knowledge, shared knowledge, theoretical knowledge accompanied by increased problem solving skills. Those who participate in clinical supervision are better able to integrate theory and practice.

Ethical debate

Practitioners become more able to recognise both personal and organisational challenges. When considering the care they gave and the actions they took, those receiving clinical supervision were more likely to ask, 'Is it right?' 'Is it safe?' 'Is it kind?'

Patient outcomes and staffing

It is difficult to conclusively demonstrate the impact that clinical supervision has on patient outcomes (White and Winstanley 2010). Having said that, those areas where clinical supervision had been implemented showed fewer complaints, lower sickness levels and a more effective use of staff education budgets.

Recently, McVey and Jones (2012) conducted a study to assess the effectiveness of clinical supervision groups and some of their findings are summarised in Box 16.4. Nurses attracted to clinical supervision are often self-confident, committed and competent; they also enjoy undertaking new challenges and practices.

Box 16.4 Benefits of clinical supervision (McVey and Jones, 2012)

Theme 1 – Developing as a professional

This includes exploring ideas and solutions, practicing psychological skills, considering more than practical/solution focussed answers and developing self-assurance.

Theme 2 – Importance of other group members

This covers ideas surrounding the helpfulness of sharing problems with other people, often from different professional backgrounds which reduces the feelings of isolation.

Theme 3 – Feeling safe

This includes the protected space offered by the groups, the non-judgemental and non-threatening attitudes of others contributing to the ability to admit to imperfections.

As with most things there is good and bad clinical supervision, one being the mirror image of the other.

Activity 16.4

Spend some time thinking about what factors would contribute to good supervision.

Whilst good supervision has a clear structure and common understanding between participants, bad supervision lacks structure and shared understanding. Good supervision has clearly defined aims and objective, agreed by all those involved, whilst in poor supervision these are confused and lack clarity. The outcome measures of good clinical supervision are stated and recognised, whilst they are often lacking in bad supervision. Confidentiality and choice are vital components of clinical supervision, their presence making the difference between the good and the bad.

Skills for supervision

Clinical supervision requires skills both for the supervisor and the supervisee.

Activity 16.5

Spend some time thinking about what skills you would look for in a clinical supervisor. What skills would you need to bring?

Box 16.5 Good and bad supervisors

Good supervisors	**Bad supervisors**
Skilled communicators	Poor communication skills
Open and honest	Closed attitudes, limited vision
Respectful and able to instil trust	Fail to develop the trust or respect of others
Maintain and ensure confidentiality	Confidentially is not ensured
Empower others	Disempower others and/or seek to control
Knowledgeable	Not knowledgeable

Bishop (2007) divides the skills for the supervisor into personal and managerial. Personal skills include being empathetic, supportive, able to facilitate reflection, open, respectful with good professional knowledge, commitment and a willingness to learn. These skills are underpinned by effective communication which includes the ability to actively listen, question appropriately and encourage. Supervisors need to be prepared to build trust so that challenge and constructive criticism can be part and parcel of the supervision process. Management skills include the ability to ensure confidentiality, act as buffer, promote accountability, organise and ensure a 'no blame culture' within the relationship (Bishop, 2007). Campbell (2006) adds knowledge to this list including knowledge about legal/ethical issues, clinical supervision strategies and the ability to help supervisees to set goals, objectives and a plan for achieving them. Driscoll (2000) noted that supervisors need to have the ability to open, what he calls the supervisory account, and be willing to learn from the process. They need to be attentive to what is going on, give and receive feedback on practice and then be able to summarise the content of the session.

Box 16.5 summarises the attributes of good and bad supervisors and as to be expected, one is the mirror image of the other.

Supervisees, on the other, hand need the ability to make sessions work for them, partly through identifying appropriate issues/topics to bring. They need to be willing to become aware of their 'self' in practice and to develop a proactive approach to solving problems. Fowler (2013) also suggests that the supervisee needs to be open to self reflection, be prepared to admit to areas of weakness and to be willing to grow and develop. Similar to supervisors, Driscoll (2000) believes that supervisees need to be prepared to receive and give feedback on practice.

Fowler (2013) rightly identifies that self-reflection and openness are not easy skills to develop and require time and practice. On the basis of his suggestion, accept the challenge offered in Activity 16.6.

Activity 16.6

Over the next week, notice your reactions each time you meet a new patient. Think about how you react – what do you think and feel? Try and identify what prompts these thoughts and feelings.

Fowler (2013) maintains that if you really commit yourself to doing this, at the end of the week, not only will you have learnt a lot about yourself, you will be convinced of the power of self-reflection.

Conclusion

In this chapter we have looked at the ways for you to have received professional support. We have considered the individuals who may help including your mentor and personal tutor, as well as the services offered by occupational health and student services. The process and benefits of clinical supervision have been discussed.

Glossary

Active listening	Listening with all the senses; fully engaged in the process.
Clinical supervision	A process whereby practice is examined in order to learn and develop.
Clinical supervision contract	An agreement entered into by those involved in clinical supervision.
Closed groups	A group that does not allow new members to join once it has formed.
Empathy	Ability to understand another person's situation from their perspective, 'putting yourself in their shoes'.
Evidenced-based care	Care which is delivered according to best evidence.
Facilitating learning	Enabling an individual to learn.
Formal learning activities	Planned learning activities such as lectures, seminars and so on.
Informal learning activities	Unplanned opportunistic learning such as talking to patients.
Mentor	A member of the clinical staff who acts as a role model for students and maybe involved with assessing their clinical competence.
'No blame culture'	Mistakes are viewed as learning opportunities and not someone's fault.
Occupational Health Department	Department which looks after the health of employees within the workplace.
Personal tutor	A member of the academic staff who provides personal and academic support.
Self-awareness	The capacity for introspection and the ability to recognise oneself as an individual separate from the environment and others.

Standards of care	The level to which care is provided.
Student services	A resource for students offering help with a range of support from financial advice to essay writing.
Supervisor	The facilitator of clinical supervision.
Supervisee	The person receiving supervision.
Work/life balance	The balance between life at work and life outside.

References

Aranda, S. (2008). The cost of caring. In: Payne, S., Seymour, J. and Ingleton, C. (eds). *Palliative Care Nursing Principles and Evidence for Practice*, 2nd edn. Maidenhead Open University Press, pp. 573–590.

Bennett, C. (2002). Making the most of mentorship. *Nursing Standard*. 17(3): 29.

Bishop, V. (1994). Clinical Supervision for an accountable profession. *Nursing Times*. 90(39): 35–37.

Bishop, V. (2006). The policy- practice divide. *Journal of Research in Nursing*. 11(3): 249–51.

Bishop, V. (2007). Literature review: clinical supervision evaluation studies. In Bishop, V. (ed.). Clinical Supervision in Practice: Some Questions, Answers and Guidelines for Professionals in Health and Social Care. Basingstoke: Palgrave Macmillan.

Bishop, V. (2008a). Clinical supervision: What is it? Why do we need it?. In: Bishop, V. (ed). *Clinical Supervision in Practice Some Questions, Answers and Guidelines for Professional in Health and Social Care*, 2nd edn. Basingstoke Palgrave Macmillan, pp. 1–26.

Bishop, V. (2008b). Clinical supervision: functions and goals. In: Bishop, V. (ed). *Clinical Supervision in Practice Some Questions, Answers and Guidelines for Professional in Health and Social Care*, 2nd edn. Basingstoke Palgrave Macmillan, pp. 27–50.

Butterworth, T. and Faugier, J. (1992). *Clinical supervision and mentorship in nursing*. London: Chapman and Hal.

Butterworth, T., Bell, L., Jackson, C. and Pajnkihar, M. (2008). Wicked spell or magic bullet? A review of the clinical supervision literature 2001-2007. *Nurse Education Today*. 28: 264–272.

Campbell, J.M. (2006). *Essentials of Clinical Supervision*. Hoboken, NJ: John Wiley & Sons Inc.

Cassedy, P. (2010). *First Steps in Clinical Supervision A Guide for Healthcare Professionals*. Maidenhead: Open University Press.

Cross, S. (2009). *Adult Teaching & Learning Developing Your Practice*. Maidenhead: McGraw Hill.

Department of Health. (1993). *Vision for the Future: The Nursing, Midwifery and Health Visiting Contribution to Health and Health Care*. London: HMSO.

Department of Health. (1994). *Clinical Supervision for the Nursing and Health Visiting Professions CNO Letter 94(5)*. London: HMSO.

Driscoll, J. (2000). *Practising Clinical Supervision A Reflective Approach*. London: Bailliere Tindall.

Faugier, J. and Butterworth, T. (1994). *Clinical Supervision: A Position Paper*. Manchester: Manchester University.

Fowler, J. (2013). Advanced practice: from staff nurse to nurse consultant. Part 4: clinical supervision. *British Journal of Nursing*. 22(4): 240.

Gopee, N. (2011). *Mentorship and Supervision in Healthcare*, 2nd edn. London: Sage.

Hawkins, P. and Shohet, R. (1989). *Supervision in the Helping Professions. An Individual, Group and Organisational Approach*. Milton Keynes: Open University Press.

Mannix, K. A., Blackburn, I. V., Garland, A., Gracie, J., Moorey, S., Reid, B., Standart, S. and Scott, J. (2006). Effectiveness of brief training in cognitive behavioural therapy techniques for palliative care practitioners. *Palliative Medicine*. 20: 579–584.

McVey, J. and Jones, T. (2012). Assessing the value of facilitated reflective practice groups. *Cancer Nursing Practice*. 11(8): 32–37.

Morton-Cooper, A. and Palmer, A. (2000). *Mentoring, Preceptorship and Clinical Supervision A guide to professional Support Roles in Clinical Practice*, 2nd edn. Abingdon: Blackwell Science.

Nursing and Midwifery Council. (2008). *Standards to Support Learning and Assessment in Practice*. London: NMC.

Proctor, B. (1986). On being a trainer: training and supervision for counselling in action. In: Hawkins, P. and Shohet, R. (eds). *Supervision in the Helping Professions*. Milton Keynes: Open University Press.

Royal College of Nursing. (2002). *Clinical Supervision in the Workplace A Guide for Occupational Health Nurse*. London: Royal College of Nursing.

Royal College of Nursing. (2011). *Spirituality in Nursing Care a Pocket Guide*. London: RCN.

United Kingdom Central Council for Nursing Midwifery and Health Visiting. (1986). *Project 2000: A New Preparation for Practice*. London: UKCC.

White, E. and Winstanley, J. (2010). A randomised controlled trial of clinical supervision: selected findings from a novel Australian attempt to establish the evidence base for causal relationships with quality of care and patient outcomes, as an informed contribution to mental health nursing practice development. *Journal of Research in Nursing*. 15(2): 151–167.

17

Learning from your practice through reflection

Introduction

Each person to whom you provide palliative care will enhance your knowledge of how to care for people with life-limiting illnesses. As you progress through your nursing, each time you meet someone with palliative care needs, you may find yourself thinking have I come across this situation before? What did I do to help patients in a similar situation? Every experience adds to our knowledge base and influences future practice. This learning can be strengthened if it is formalised through the process of reflective practice. Reflection is vital when providing palliative care for patients; it helps you to understand their situation, their perspectives and their needs. Reflection will also help you to understand your own responses to individual patient situations. This chapter will look at the place of reflective practice in palliative care and how it might benefit you.

Fundamentals of Palliative Care for Student Nurses, First Edition. Megan Rosser and Helen C. Walsh.

Companion website: www.wiley.com/go/rosser_walsh/fundamentals_of_palliative_care

Learning outcomes

At the end of the chapter you will be able to

- describe reflective practice;
- understand reflection as a learning strategy;
- discuss some of the reflective practice models available;
- consider how reflective practice can help your practice and development.

Reflection helps us to learn from experience in order to make sense of complex situations. Its origins can be attributed to the Greek philosopher, Aristotle who emphasised the importance of reflecting in the 'real world' in order to develop the experience of it. Perhaps the first modern influential advocate of reflection is the educationalist and philosopher, John Dewey. Dewey (1938) saw reflection as thinking with a purpose, in order to learn from our actions, whilst acknowledging the role of emotions and feelings as part of the process as well as the consequences of our actions.

Within professional education, Donald Schon (1983) has been influential in the development of reflection differentiating between 'reflection in action' and 'reflection on action'. Reflective practice was acknowledged by Schon as a process that could develop the professional knowledge of practitioners through encouraging them to think critically about what they do in practice, how they use their knowledge to influence practice and how practice can develop as a result of that knowledge.

Nowadays, reflection and reflective practice are regarded by many as essential attributes of competent health care professionals, being able to learn from your practice is vital in ensuring competence across your working life (Mann *et al.*, 2009). As a student nurse you may be quite familiar with the concepts of reflection, reflective learning and reflective practice as they have been part of most nursing curricula for many years now and are endorsed by the NMC as fundamental skills required of nursing students (NMC, 2008).

Reflection, reflective learning and reflective practice all help us to learn from experience, to further our understanding and to inform our practice therefore it is important to have an understanding of each.

Activity 17.1

Write a description of reflection, reflective practice and reflective learning and compare them to the descriptions below.

Reflection is a way of looking at practice from a number of different angles. Reflection informs both reflective practice and reflective learning.

Reflective practice is about learning from experience and developing our practice as a consequence.

Reflective learning is the process of learning from experiences, reconsidering our existing knowledge and adding this new learning to our knowledge in order to inform our practice.

Jasper and Rosser (2013)

Reflection enables a reflective practitioner to review an incident from practice from as many angles as possible in order to work out:

- what happened?
- what the practitioner thought or felt at the time?
- why they thought or felt that?
- who else was involved?
- what the others might have thought and felt?

This helps the practitioner to understand the situation and the people involved more deeply (Bolton, 2010).

Reflection and reflective learning are active processes, they do not just happen, we have to find time to think about our practice in a structured way in order to understand it better and to learn from it. Reflection may be undertaken as a solitary activity through reflective writing, possibly in a reflective diary, or as a one to one discussion with a mentor or supervisor, or in a group engaging in reflective practice or clinical supervision.

Leading on from reflective learning, reflective practice has three components (Jasper and Rosser, 2013):

- the experience upon which to reflect;
- the process of reflection and the learning that arises from that reflection;
- the action taken as a result of the learning.

Action taken as a result of the learning is the crux of reflective practice, if no action is taken as the result of reflective learning then there is no impact on practice. Whilst the reflection may have enlightened you and increased your understanding of a situation it is meaningless in terms of reflective practice.

Activity 17.2

Think about how reflection, reflective learning and reflective practice have influenced your development to date.

It might help to think about a critical incident in your experience as a student so far (either in University or in practice) and consider the following:

Why was it important to you?

What did you learn from it?

Types of reflection

Schon (1983) identified two main types of reflection.

Reflection in action

This reflection occurs whilst a problem is being addressed; it helps us to complete a task or an action, to change what we are doing whilst we are doing it. We tend to use reflection in action when things are not going the way we expected them to, or our normal actions are not working and we need to think of alternative actions. Professionals demonstrate the ability to 'think what they are doing while they are doing it'. Professionals who reflect in action have the ability to think on their feet and apply previous experience to a situation in order to solve the problem, or at least alleviate it.

A nursing example of this could be communicating with a patient who is contemplating the impact of their illness on their future, and having to frame questions in response to what patients say; thinking about the best way to communicate in order to keep the conversation going. If a patient becomes very distressed, how to respond to them? Communicating with dying patients and families most definitely requires the ability to think on your feet as it is not always possible to anticipate how such a conversation is going to go. Although no two such conversations are ever identical there will be principles of communication that the nurse is aware of, partly from what she has been taught and also from experiences of similar conversations with previous patients.

Activity 17.3

Think about a patient interaction/intervention when you used reflection in action. It might be something as simple but vital as encouraging a reluctant patient to eat or drink.

Did you have to change the way you approached the patient?
How did you get the patient to take the food or fluid?
What knowledge and/or previous experience did you use to guide your interaction with your patient?
Have you previously had the experience of feeding patients who were not interested?
Have you practised feeding your student colleagues in college before going on to the ward and therefore knew some different approaches to take?
Have you had any personal experience of trying to encourage someone to eat?

Think about these things in relation to an activity you have been involved in, with a patient where you had to make a decision about what to do whilst doing it.

Reflection on action

This reflection occurs after an event and is consciously undertaken in order to discover more about the situation, gain a deeper understanding of it and to learn from it. Reflection on action is retrospective; it may follow a particular framework and is often documented or shared with colleagues. Learning from practice may generate new clinical knowledge and ultimately add to the evidence base for nursing. Skills required for effective reflection on action include

- recall;
- analysis;
- flexibility and the ability to see things from different perspectives;
- interpretation;
- being open minded;
- willingness to put aside strong opinions and to learn new knowledge;
- ability to apply new knowledge to practice.

There is a tendency for many nurses to use reflection on action following events that have not gone as well as hoped. It is equally good practice to use it to celebrate good experiences so that we know what to do the next time. When providing palliative nursing care you could chose to use reflection on action after a patient died peacefully, free from pain or any other troublesome symptoms, in the place of their choice, surrounded by people of their choice. Reflection on action would help you understand why things went so well for the patient and their family and to establish what was it that made it a particularly 'good death?'

Anticipatory reflection

A third type of reflection has been suggested by Van Manen (1991) and Greenwood (1993). Van Manen calls it anticipatory reflection whilst Greenwood coined the phrase reflection before action. The purpose of this type of action is to enable practitioners to plan an intervention or interaction and anticipate the consequences of that action. Past experience is also taken into account when using anticipatory reflection.

Nurses use this approach to reflection, when planning care for their patients. A community nurse visiting a patient for the first time may use anticipatory reflection when she is thinking about how she will conduct the assessment, focussing on issues that she anticipates the patient will bring up and thinking about how the visit will go. Anticipatory reflection enables the nurse to plan her care to a degree, conversely if things do not go the way she anticipates, she may find herself reflecting in action to ensure that the assessment goes as well as possible.

Why use reflective practice?

Activity 17.4

What do you think the benefits of reflective practice might be and for whom?

Compare your answers to those listed in Table 17.1.

There are many benefits for you as an individual. Continually developing your knowledge and practice through reflection prevents you from becoming stuck in your ways. It encourages you to question practice and to look for alternative ways of caring for patients. Reflection also gives you the opportunity to apply what you learn in the classroom to your clinical practice areas, allowing you to test out your knowledge in order to consolidate your learning and develop your practice.

When professionals engage in reflective practice they start to incorporate evidence based nursing care and develop it further to inform their practice, this increases the likelihood of the provision of safe, individualised, quality patient care. This in turn has positive benefits for the employing organisation in terms of clinical reputation and staff satisfaction.

Finally the nursing profession itself benefits from continual development of nursing knowledge and the articulation of the nursing contribution in the constantly changing health care environment.

Reflection therefore offers a valuable way to learn from experience, to gain new knowledge and to challenge practice. It offers an opportunity to critically reflect on how practice events and situations are affecting us as individuals and conversely how we as individuals are affecting practice.

Table 17.1 The benefits of reflective practice

Who benefits?	Benefits
You	• Affirms your own good practice. • Ensures you are giving evidence-based care rather than routine care. • Focuses on your patients as individuals. • Maximises your learning opportunities. – Identifies shortfalls in your knowledge and skills. – Identifies your learning needs. • Continually develops your knowledge base and practice.
Your patients	• Receive a better quality of care. • Individualised and evidence-based care derived from their particular needs. • Better standards of patient safety. • Improved decision making. • A reduction in the number of adverse patient incidents (such as drug errors, falls). • More confidence in professional practitioners.
Your employer	• A good reputation for professional practice. • Higher standards and quality of care. • Better recruitment and retention. • A multi-skilled workforce • Effective appraisal mechanisms, resulting in: – training and development needs – reduced adverse patient 'incidents'; – less litigation.
Your profession	• Increased public confidence. • Increased inter-professional parity. • Raised professional profile and standing. • Developing the nursing knowledge base. • Recognition of nursing specific skills. • Recognition of the unique contribution that nursing makes to patient care.

Jasper and Rosser (2013)

Starting your reflective practice

Reflection can be undertaken in three different arenas and whilst the process and requisite skills are very similar, they present different opportunities and challenges. The arenas are alone, in groups and for academic assessment.

Reflecting by ourselves

When an incident or experience affects us, either positively or negatively, we may be prompted to reflect on it in order to learn from that experience. This is a very personal activity; it can involve writing things down, using a reflective framework to give structure or merely thinking critically about the event. Writing things down can be cathartic as well as providing a record which can be revisited at a future date. Indeed Tate (2013) describes learning to write reflectively as the key skill needed in order to learn from the reflective process. As a nursing student you will probably have been encouraged to maintain a reflective journal, thus keeping a record of learning and development. Whilst Bolton (2010) describes a journal as a diary with a purpose, it can also help to develop self-awareness (Billington, 2013). Tate (2013) prefers the term 'personal' rather than 'reflective' to describe the journal for a number of reasons including the fact that it is personal to the writer and avoids any potential barriers resulting from the term 'reflective'.

Reflecting by ourselves on something that is important to us is often exciting as we are totally free to go wherever our thoughts lead us, often identifying things that we had never recognised or acknowledged before. However it requires a good deal of honesty and self-awareness. Without these attributes, we could be overcritical or become complacent, missing opportunities to recognise our strengths or areas which need development. It is also important to remember that reflection is not just about thinking, it is also about actions which follow on from these thoughts. When reflecting alone, it is possible for the action part to be forgotten.

Reflecting with others

This is one way of overcoming some of the drawbacks of reflecting by ourselves. We can reflect with a single colleague or friend, with peers or join a reflective group. The effectiveness of group reflection depends on the group and the reasons why it has been established. For example, groups maybe informal or structured, hierarchical or democratic, single or multidisciplinary (Carter, 2013). As long as the structure of the group suits its purpose, which is acknowledged by all members, then each is as effective as another.

Reflection for academic assessment

Most nurses will at some point in their education and development be asked to write a reflective assignment using a designated framework. Some argue that using a framework restricts freedom of thought, reflection and the flow of the writing. Approaching the task with an open mindset and a willingness to learn from the process can be beneficial.

The first stage involves choosing the focus of the reflection. Some nurses will find this very easy to do whilst others struggle a little. When choosing what to reflect upon it may be helpful to use the acronym SODA (Jasper and Rosser, 2013) to help you select an experience. Experiences selected for reflection should be:

Significant	It stands out for you for some reason.
Outcome	There needs to have been some development for you.
Describable	It can de described in its entirety accurately and without breeching confidentiality.
Action	It resulted in some action being taken.

Activity 17.5

Think of an interaction you have had with a palliative care patient and see if it fulfils all the criteria of SODA.

Write down how it fulfils each criterion.

An example may be the first time you spent time sitting, listening and talking with a patient about how they feel about their disease and the impact it has on their life. This is not a particularly easy situation to find yourself in, so it may well be beneficial to reflect upon your experience.

Significant	It was the first time you had had such a conversation with a patient. It was emotional and you found it quite difficult to stay and listen. It made you think about the essay on communication you were working on.
Outcome	It made you think about how you could be more prepared for listening to other patients. It made you feel you did not know enough about communicating with dying patients. It made you realise you wanted to know more about how that disease might progress and the impact that would have on your patient and his family. It made you wonder why you found it so hard.
Describable	It was a conversation that occurred last week and lasted for 15 min. You were able to recall the content of the conversation.
Action	You went away and read more about communicating with patients with short prognoses. You went away and read more about the disease and its progression. You spoke to your mentor about how you might have handled it differently.

Models of reflection

Having decided on the subject of your reflection you need to find a model or framework that will help guide your reflection. Whilst experienced and proficient reflective practitioners may not use a formal model to guide their reflection, novice reflectors will probably find that a model or framework provides structure for an unfamiliar activity. Most models consist of a series of cue questions or a checklist for the reflective practitioner to work through in order to facilitate experiential learning. Regardless of whether or not a framework is used for reflection a reflective practitioner needs to possess certain skills in order to be able to reflect effectively. These are shown in Box 17.1.

Perhaps the reflective models most commonly used in nurse education are those developed by Gibbs (1988) and Johns (2010).

Gibbs (1988) model was developed to help student teachers develop their teaching skills and as such is an educationally driven model as opposed to practice driven. It is criticised by some for failing to show the application of new knowledge to practice. Its final stage is purely a consideration of what you would do if you found yourself in the same situation again. It does

Box 17.1 Skills of reflection

- Self-awareness – the ability to be able to analyse feelings in order to explore the significance of a situation or experience.
- Description – the ability to recognise and accurately remember relevant features of a particular situation or experience.
- Critical analysis – being able to examine the components of the situation or experience, recognising existing knowledge, challenging assumptions, imagining and exploring alternatives.
- Synthesis – the ability to integrate new knowledge with existing knowledge in a creative way in order to solve problems or plan future actions.
- Evaluation – the ability to judge the value of something.

Bulman (2013)

not require you to take action in order to change practice. Despite its critics it is a model chosen by many students for its apparent simplicity and ease of application. It comprises six stages – see Figure 17.1.

Johns' model of structured reflection was designed specifically to facilitate reflection on practice. It aims to facilitate deeper understanding of a clinical event from a variety of perspectives in order to explicate the underpinning nursing knowledge. It is based upon Carper's ways of knowing (1978) which proposed that there were different kinds of knowledge that were equally important in understanding nursing.

Empirical knowledge – that drawn from the nursing knowledge and theories, some of which you are taught during your education – the science of nursing.

Aesthetic knowledge – the artistry of nursing – the subjective intuitive knowledge that enables practitioners to understand the situation they find themselves in and respond instinctively to patients as individuals. This body of knowledge develops with experience.

Personal knowledge – develops from self-awareness of how the nurse responds to her patients and how she uses herself within the therapeutic relationship.

Ethical knowledge – is knowledge that is derived from ethical and moral principles which guide practice.

Activity 17.6

Think about how these kinds of knowledge can inform palliative care nursing:

Empirical The theoretical knowledge about disease processes, pain and symptom management, communication theories, bereavement theories.

Aesthetic The art of nursing, expert nursing, understanding and accompanying the patient journey.

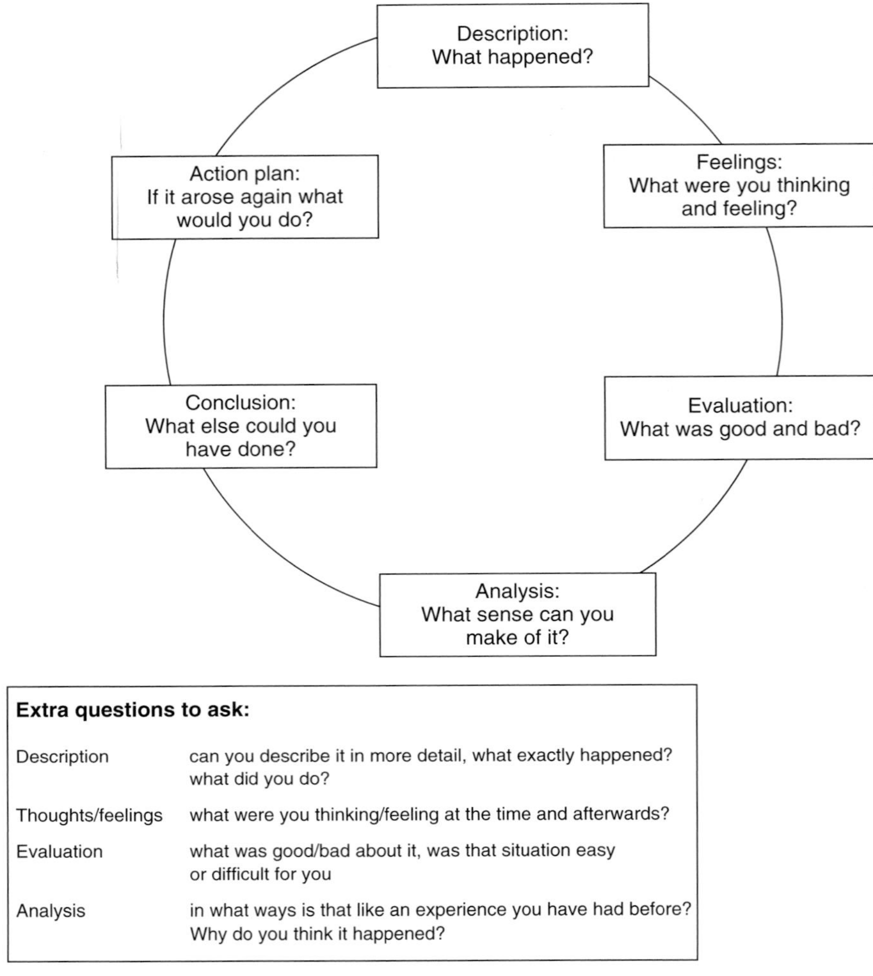

Figure 17.1 Gibbs reflective cycle (1988).

Personal	How you act and respond to your patients, what impact if has on you and how that influences your ability to provide appropriate nursing care.
Ethical	Awareness of the ethical and moral challenges towards the end of life such as decisions around treatment, euthanasia and resuscitation.

At a glance it appears that Carper's ways of knowing are all extremely applicable to palliative care, therefore you may well find Johns' model of structured reflection an invaluable guide for your initial reflections. Johns has refined his model over many years and it incorporates many facets in additions to Carper's ways of knowing, see Box 17.2.

A model that is gaining popularity in nursing is Borton's (1970) three step reflective framework. Like Gibbs' model it was initially rooted in educational development but has been adopted by

Box 17.2 Johns' Model for Structured Reflection

1. Bring the mind home.
2. Write a description of an experience that seems significant in some way.
3. What issues seem significant to pay attention to?
4. How were the others feeling and what made them feel that way?
5. How was I feeling and what made me feel that way?
6. What was I trying to achieve and did I respond effectively?
7. What were the consequences of my actions on the patient, others and myself?
8. What factors influenced the way I was thinking, feeling or responding?
9. What knowledge did or might have informed me?
10. To what extent did I act for the best and in tune with my values?
11. How did this situation connect with previous experiences?
12. How might I reframe the situation and respond more effectively given this situation again?
13. What would be the consequences of alternative actions for the patient, others and myself?
14. What factors might constrain me from responding differently?
15. How do I now feel about this experience?
16. Am I now more able to support myself and others better as a consequence?
17. What insights do I draw towards self-realisation?

Johns' (2010 p. 36)

practitioners in other professions to guide their reflections. It asks the practitioner three very simple questions:

- What?
- So what?
- Now what?

The 'what?' requires the practitioner to identify a significant event, to describe it and to identify the main issues arising from that event. The 'so what?' then enables the practitioner to reflect on action by analysing and evaluating the main points arising from the 'what?'. The 'now what?' helps us to consider alternative courses of action and decide what we need to do next. Rolfe (2011) have expanded Borton's framework by developing cue questions for each stage.

As you can see there is a pattern emerging, regardless of which model you use there are similar stages for you to go through during your reflection. Jasper (2013) has identified them as below:

Stage one: selecting a critical incident to reflect on.
Stage two: observing and describing the experience.
Stage three: analysing the experience.
Stage four: interpreting the experience.
Stage five: exploring alternatives.
Stage six: framing action.

Activity 17.7

Returning to the incident you identified as appropriate to reflect upon, have a go reflecting upon the incident using the reflective frameworks/models presented here.

Which did you prefer and why?

It is good to have a go at using a number of reflective models as one model will not suit all of us. Practitioners will tend to eventually find one model that they prefer. It is good practice to use a model to help you discover and develop your skills of reflective practice. Experienced reflective practitioners have become skilled at fulfilling all stages of the reflective process and may not rely on the structure of a model or framework to guide their reflections, preferring to use their own approach. You may well reach this point given time and practice. If you did not find any of the models from this chapter easy to use there are a number of other models you might like to look at, for instance Holm and Stephenson (1994), Taylor (2006, 2010) and Fish *et al.* (1991)

Conclusion

You need to work at developing the skills of a reflective practitioner. Reflective practice is invaluable in palliative care nursing as it is a clinical area that can be fraught with many challenges. Challenges may arise at a clinical level when trying to get a patient's symptoms under control or an emotional level when you are caring for people and families who are confronting a number of losses in a shortened life. The ethical challenges are getting increasingly complex with the advances in medical care. Caring for dying patients and their families comes at a cost to you. Using reflective practice will enable you to understand your responses to the numerous challenges of palliative care situations you experience and to identify what you have to do in order to look after yourself. It will also help you identify what you need to learn in order to care for your palliative care patients to the best of your ability.

Reflective practice will enable you to develop throughout your nurse education and as you progress through your nursing career. It will ensure that your practice remains current and evidence based and will encourage you to challenge the areas of routine care to ensure that patient care is of the highest standard possible.

Glossary

Anticipatory reflection — Undertaken before an event to enable practitioners to plan an intervention or interaction and anticipate the consequences of that action.

Reflection — Is a way of looking at practice from a number of different angles.

Reflective learning — The process of learning from experiences, reconsidering our existing knowledge and adding this new learning to our knowledge in order to inform our practice.

Reflective practice	Learning from experience and developing our practice as a consequence.
Reflection in action	Occurs whilst a problem is being addressed or a situation occurring.
Reflection on action	Occurs after an event and is consciously undertaken in order to learn from it.

References

Billington, T. (2013). Promoting self-awareness through reflective practice. *British Journal of Nursing*. 22(1): 45.

Bolton, G. (2010). *Reflective Practice – Writing and Professional Development*, 3rd edn. London: Sage.

Borton, T. (1970). *Reach, Touch and Teach*. London: Hutchinson.

Bulman, C. (2013). Getting started on a journey with reflection. In: Bulman, C. and Schutz, S. (eds). *Reflective Practice in Nursing*, 5th edn. Chichester: John Wiley & Sons, Ltd, pp. 1–22.

Carper, B.A. (1978). Fundamental patterns of knowing in nursing. *Advances in Nursing Science*. 1(1): 13–24.

Carter, B. (2013). Reflecting in groups. In: Bulman, C. and Schutz, S. (eds). *Reflective Practice in Nursing*, 5th edn. Chichester: John Wiley & Sons, Ltd, pp. 93–120.

Dewey J. (1938). *Experience and Education*. New York: Macmillan.

Fish, D., Twinn, S. and Purr, B. (1991). *Promoting Reflection: Improving the Supervision of Practice in Health Visiting and Initial Teacher Training*. London: West London Institute of Higher Education.

Gibbs, G. (1988). *Learning by Doing. A Guide to Teaching and Learning Methods*. Oxford: Further Education Unit, Oxford Polytechnic.

Greenwood, J. (1993). Some considerations concerning practice and feedback in nursing education. *Journal of Advanced Nursing*. 18: 1999–2002.

Holm, D. and Stephenson, S. (1994). Reflection – a student's perspective. In: Palmer, A., Burns, S. and Bulman, C. (eds). *Reflective Practice in Nursing*. Oxford: Blackwell Publishing.

Jasper, M. (2013). *Beginning Reflective Practice*, 2nd edn. Cheltenham: Nelson Thrones.

Jasper, M. and Rosser, M. (2013). Reflection and reflective practice. In: Jasper, M., Rosser, M. and Mooney, G. (eds). *Professional Development, Reflection and Decision Making in Nursing and Healthcare*. Oxford: John Wiley & Sons, Ltd.

Johns, C. (2010) Constructing the reflexive narrative. In: Johns, C. (ed). *Guided Reflection: A Narrative Approach to Advancing Professional Practice*, 2nd edn. Oxford: Wiley-Blackwell.

Mann, K., Gordon, J. and MacLeod, A. (2009). Reflection and reflective practice in health professions education: a systematic review. *Advances in Health Science Education*. 14: 595–621.

Nursing and Midwifery Council. (2008) *Standards to Support Learning and Assessment in Practice*. London: NMC.

Rolfe, G. (2011). Models and frameworks for critical reflection. In: Rolfe, G., Jasper, M. and Freshwater, D. (eds). *Critical Reflection in Practice: Generating Knowledge for Care*, 2nd edn. Basingstoke: Palgrave Macmillan.

Schon, D.A. (1983). *The Reflective Practitioner: How Professionals Think in Action*. Aldershot: Arena.

Tate, S. (2013). Writing to learn: writing reflectively. In: Bulman, C. and Schutz, S. (eds). *Reflective Practice in Nursing*, 5th edn. Chichester: John Wiley & Sons, Ltd, pp. 53–92.

Taylor, B.J. (2006). *Reflective Practice for Healthcare Professionals*, 2nd edn. Maidenhead: Open University Press.

Taylor, B.J. (2010). *Reflective Practice for Healthcare Professionals*, 3rd edn. Maidenhead: Open University Press.

Van Manen, M. (1991). Reflectivity and the pedagogical moment: the normativity of pedagogical thinking and acting. *Journal of Curriculum Studies*. 23: 507–536.

Index

Fundamentals of Palliative Care for Student Nurses, First Edition. Megan Rosser and Helen C. Walsh.